T0128101

THE SMART GIRL'S GUIDE TO THE G-SPOT

THE SMART GIRL'S GUIDE TO THE G-SPOT

VIOLET BLUE

FOREWORD BY JESSE BERING

CLEiS
PRESS

Published in the United States by Cleis Press Inc., 2246 Sixth St., Berkeley, CA 94710.

Printed in the United States.
Cover design: Scott Idleman/Blink
Cover photograph: momentimages
Text design: Karen Quigg
Second Edition.
10 9 8 7 6 5 4 3 2 1

Trade paper ISBN: 978-1-57344-780-5
E-book ISBN: 978-1-57344-783-6

Library of Congress Cataloging-in-Publication Data is available.

contents

foreword
by jesse bering

When I was in the ninth grade, ninety pounds when wet, secretly gay, and prone to unbidden orgasms at the banal tickles of the atmosphere, I placed in my "girlfriend's" palm a pornographic note so riddled with perversions that if ever that voice in the back of her head telling her that my lust burned not for her, but rather for her older brother, were to burst suddenly into her consciousness, the memory of this debauched ode would reel her back to doubt. It would be dishonest to say that I recall all the absurdly obscene things the letter contained, but there was almost certainly a line about my hope of flossing with her pubic hair after smearing her buttocks with my cream. (In reality, I'd have run for my life if she actually welcomed this scene.)

Soon, the two of us would be called down to the vice principal's office, where a raft of sunlight set us all afloat on a sober discussion about the seriousness of my written offense, which had found its way into his hands. "Are you afraid of him?" said the middle-aged man to my fake girlfriend, nodding at me without looking at me, "I mean, there are some pretty disturbing things in this letter."

What she snapped back at him made me fall madly in love with her. "Afraid?" she fired back. "How sad. Don't you ever say anything like that anymore to your wife?"

Now I'm all grown up and a gay psychologist, and I can talk about penises without pretending to like pussies. Actually, it's not that I *don't* like them—I just don't go into them in my private life. I do see female ejaculation as an enormously fascinating subject matter that has largely escaped serious scientific inquiry, particularly from an evolutionary perspective. This is all the more puzzling given that female ejaculation, which is usually defined as the expulsion of a significant amount of fluid around the time of orgasm—estimates range from, on average, 3 to 50 ml (about 10 teaspoons)—is a topic that was first described by scholars around 2,000 years ago.

The fourth century Taoist text, "Secret Instructions Concerning the Jade Chamber," for example, written for the enterprising man in the art of satisfying a woman in bed, suggested that he decipher the following "five signs" of feminine arousal accordingly:

1. "reddened face" = "she wants to make love with you"
2. "breasts hard and nose perspiring" = "she wants you to insert your penis"
3. "throat dry and saliva blocked" = "she is very stimulated and excited"
4. "slippery vagina" = "she wants to have her orgasm soon"
5. "the genitals transmit fluid" = "she has already been satisfied"

I wouldn't recommend any man follow these secret instructions today; citing number two in your defense that, say, some woman with a sweaty nose wanted you to insert your penis into her isn't likely to hold up in a court of law. But the fact that this ancient text distinguishes between "slippery vagina" and "the genitals transmit fluid," means that even the ancients knew of female ejaculation. Likewise, the *Kamasutra*, which dates to 200-400 A.D., speaks of "female semen" that "falls continually." In the West, even Aristotle had something to say about female discharge during sexual intercourse, which, he pointed out, "far exceeds" the seminal emission of the man. He also noted—and it's tempting to speculate about just how he came to this conclusion—that female ejaculation tends to be "found in those who are fair-skinned and of a feminine type generally, but not in those who are dark and of masculine appearance." Astounding that it wasn't until 1982 that female ejaculate was first analyzed in terms of its chemical properties. And guess what—it wasn't urine!

It's as though Aristotle was prognosticating in his mind's eye our own Violet Blue—the "the fair-skinned, feminine type" with the liberated vulva. I don't know what ever happened to that clever girl from high school who served so generously as my beard, but I imagine she's probably something like Violet—the brilliantly naughty schoolgirl grown up, unrepentantly sexual, fearlessly playful, always up for a mind-fuck with her gay male friends, and a ravenous brain matched only by an even more ravenous G-spot. So sit back, slide your hands down there, and let Violet push your buttons.

introduction:
thoughts on becoming
supreme master overlord
of your g-spot

The G-spot is not a riddle wrapped in a mystery inside an enigma. It is a place in your body. In my body. It's a real, tangible thing, like my breasts and your clitoris, and you can even see it. But for some reason, lots of people seem to think the G-spot is a myth. Or a rumor. Or something only for the granola-and-Birkenstocks crowd, who call it the "goddess spot" and claim we tap into our "inner wisdom" when we go hunting around for it. No— it's a real thing, and it makes you come, hard, period. No deep wisdom, soul-searching or goddess worship necessary. But a little knowledge helps.

That's why I had to write this G-spot guide for smart girls like me. There are way, way too many guys online who think that watching porn or reading other people's websites gives them the knowl-

edge to spout off about what is and isn't up with
the G-spot and female ejaculation—often getting
their facts wrong in horrifyingly shaming ways.
And the only books I could find out there were either piecemeal, dated, or intended for an audience
of women who wanted a spiritual experience—
when all I wanted was to figure out how to get off.
None of these books or websites spoke to me, and
some of them offended and scared me. It seemed like
no one could just talk about the G-spot in plain, even
fun, terms. It either got glossed over in explaining
a mystery of some kind, or it had to be cloaked in
feminist reclaiming or Mother Earth context, as if
the people doing the explaining had to give the G-
spot some kind of extra validation to make it okay
to talk about in the first place. Rather than turning
me on and making me want to get out the lube, this
approach has the same effect as a Thorazine dart. It
puts any wild animal—or horny smart girl—to sleep.

I want to encourage you to think of this volume
not just as a G-spot guide for smart girls, but also
as a call to arms for girls who want to be a little
bit more fierce about their sexuality. We're not reclaiming the G-spot here; we're making plans for
orgasmic lawlessness. We're not searching for a
mythical magic button buried somewhere in our
pussies; we're constructing a doomsday device in

the basement. We're not worried that we might pee ourselves with pleasure (because we won't); we're ramping up to feel really, really good about our bad selves. It's like that.

This book has attitude, and a lot of helpful information to back it up. In the first chapter you'll find out what the big deal is about the G-spot, what's real and what's not, and why the G-spot has such an annoying name. Next, in chapter 2 you'll get your map to the Batcave (a G-spot anatomy lesson); in chapter 3 you'll find out how to activate your G-spot/orgasm doomsday device by learning how to stimulate it, how it feels, and all the essentials on how to proceed, including toys and techniques. In chapter 4 you'll learn how to share your new toy with a lover (including G-spot-centric sexual positions). In chapter 5, female ejaculation is explained and demystified, with lots of specific troubleshooting tips. After that, if you're ready for more, you'll find a chapter on intensifying your G-spot experience with anal, oral, S/M and fisting. Finally, there's a huge resource chapter with further reading, online shopping recommendations and safer sex info.

Interleaved with the informational text you'll also find four apt erotic stories by Alison Tyler that bring to life both the real-time exploration of this critical erotic zone and the pleasurable feelings, bodily and emotional, it can create.

So take a deep breath, leave the granola and disinformation behind, and get ready to come like a crazed hyena.

Violet Blue

get smart

The clitoris may be our smug little mistress of gratification, pure in orgasmic purpose within her princess seat atop the female pleasure system. But girls who've taken their erotic explorations further on into G-spot territory know that the clitoris is but a sweet sentry to the intense pleasure that lies within. A girl who enjoys G-spot play knows that when her clit stands at attention, the fun has only just begun. A skilled pair of slick fingers, a smooth and firm sex toy, or even a carefully angled hot cock or slippery fist can topple her clit's prim orgasms with thigh-quaking G-spot explosions that leave her sweaty and wild-eyed, clit twitching in empathy.

The sensation of a G-spot orgasm is like no other; from clitoral stimulation to anal orgasm, nothing can compare. G-spot pleasure leaves gluteal muscles

deliciously sore, makes the dogs howl and cats run
for cover, ruins bedsheets and blowouts alike, and
may even contribute to global warming. Best of all,
as the saying goes, you can't have just one. You can
have *lots*. Think of it as being like trading up your
six-shooter for a semiautomatic.

What's the Big Deal?

You might be wondering what all the G-spot noise
is about. Maybe you have your own style(s) of bringing yourself to orgasm—say with fingers, sex toys
or a friend—using clitoral and/or vaginal techniques
that are tried and true. Perhaps you have experienced
an unusual or unexpected kind of orgasm, and are
wondering if maybe it was a G-spot orgasm. It could
be that there's a way you like to get off that you think
might just be G-spot related, but aren't quite sure.
Maybe a lover wants you to try, or wants to help you
"find" your G-spot. Or you're hearing all this great
stuff about the G-spot, and want to know what the
big deal is anyway.

  If you already have an orgasmic style that you like,
you might be kind of curious about G-spot play but
don't know if you want to change what already is
reliable and feels good. That's okay—because even
if this is true and you have a lover who wants to

explore your G-spot (or you're just a *little* curious),
playing with your G-spot can be thought of as a pleasure experiment. Your G-spot is there to play with
as you like, and if you don't like it, no big deal.
Experiment concluded, hang up the lab coat.

Seeing all the magazine articles and endless G-spot
promotions and G-spot-related toys on sex toy
websites (especially the women-centric ones) this
might seem to you like a lot of hype at first. You may
have a friend who really likes G-spot play—and
sounds like a newly brainwashed member of a cult
when she talks about it. Another friend may tell a
tale of G-spot discomfort and abandoned pleasure-
seeking. It's hard to find a middle ground, and that's
because G-spot orgasms can be pretty powerful, with
a lot of strong accompanying sensations, and that's
not always for everyone.

Not every girl wants to join a sex cult, even with
a membership of one. But between the two extremes
of rabid G-spot orgasm devotion and dislike for the
sensations is a huge playing field where a girl can
experiment with G-spot stimulation like any other
sex toy in her bag. Think of it as having a few different delicious treats to choose among each time you
want to indulge yourself; you don't have to just have
the same slice of pie every night (even if the pie is
always really yummy).

Your G-spot is another way to make yourself feel good, in addition to all the other ways you already know. And for many women, adding G-spot play to their sexual repertoire takes their sex lives and cranks up the pleasure, adding a new option for orgasms, making sex more intense, and bringing diversity to the range of sex they already enjoy. It's also fun to have a new sex toy to share with a lover—one that comes in your own personal factory design.

What the G-Spot Is

Plainly put, the G-spot is an area just inside your vagina, which, when you're turned on, may feel really good to rub or massage. It may even feel so good you have an orgasm from that type of stimulation alone. About one to two inches inside and on the front (belly button side) of your vaginal canal is the route through which urine leaves your body—your urethra. The urethra is a little channel between your bladder and the outside world, and it's surrounded with erectile tissue (like that in a penis) and about forty glands and ducts that all respond pleasurably to stimulation. This is the urethral sponge. In some women, stimulation of the G-spot to orgasm is accompanied by an expulsion of fluid from the glands and ducts in the sponge, in a powerfully pleasurable (and sometimes very wet) female ejaculation. In many women, it's the urethra, or the area right around it, that responds best to stimulation.

What the G-Spot Isn't

First of all, it's not a magic button, which, once you find and press it, delivers unending waves of instant orgasms. Over the past few decades, magazine articles, online sex commerce sites, and even porn have all made the G-spot seem like the pot of gold at the end of the female orgasmic rainbow—as if you could just find it and one touch would send your eyes rolling skyward and make you come like a crazed banshee. Like most end-of-the-rainbow fables, the G-spot-as-instant-orgasm-trigger story simply isn't true. The problem is that people like to shorthand anything sexual in our culture, and it's a much better sound bite to liken its activation to flipping a switch than it is to explain the plain truths about G-spot orgasms. The truth is, G-spot stimulation to orgasm can be shown and explained pretty easily, but the details are often too explicitly sexual for the producers of most entertainment and sales outlets—in their minds, it's way more palatable to advertisers and nervous shoppers for someone to say "press it and orgasm," than "put something hard in your vagina, find the spot, jack off, and *come.*"

The Male G-Spot

In books, online, and in sexual how-to videos, you'll find that people like to use the words G-spot and prostate interchangeably when referring to both areas. The prostate gland is located at just about the center of the male urogenital system, inside the perineal wall; it can be stimulated directly by massaging one to two inches inside the anus, toward the front of a man's body. Alternately rebuked, reviled, redeemed, and romanced, this little gland manages to make headlines. Sometimes the attention is conflicted: the gland makes prostatic fluid for carrying virile semen, making the man "a man"; it also makes orgasm outrageously powerful but requires access through anal penetration, challenging some people's definition of "a man." The prostate (aka the male G-spot) is a gland that is best stimulated through anal penetration. The G-spot (aka the female prostate) is a bundle of nerves, tiny glands and erectile tissue best stimulated through vaginal penetration. Different animals, but both like to be petted.

Another thing the G-spot isn't: inaccessible. It's not high up in some unreachable place, in your deep dark mysterious cave. The vagina ceased to be a mystery about forty years ago, and I find it ridiculous that some people (especially online) still say that the G-spot might be hard to find. Let's oversimplify for a moment with a hands-on tutorial that requires no hands at all. To get an idea where to find the spot, go to the toilet, pee, and see where it comes from. Ding! There's the map to your buried treasure; this is the urethral opening, the outside indicator of your G-spot's underground hideout. Don't pay attention to anyone who says that it might be difficult to find. (Or that you may lose track of it; hilariously, some pundits have suggested that it travels, or can get "lost," not unlike Hippocrates' not-so-adorable decrees that the uterus wandered freely about a woman's body should it become discontented or angry. It makes my uterus angry enough to take a walk just thinking about such misinformation.) You don't need a flashlight, a hand mirror or familiarity with self-examination to find it. But if you want to use any of those tools, great; otherwise you can locate and stimulate it with your fingers, a sex toy or a lover's penis (or strap-on). Again, having a G-spot (or not) is not a roll of the dice—everyone has a urethra, otherwise they'd never be able to pee.

You don't have to be on an inner journey to play with it. The G-spot is for every woman, not just ones who seek transcendent wisdom through personal sexual exploration. It's not a spiritual gateway (though some women say that sometimes G-spot orgasms can be cosmic in scale), nor do you need to be enlightened to find it. As with anything sexual, you'll be interested in the G-spot for any number of reasons, and how you play with it and experiment with it will change and evolve over time. Your attitude and techniques, preferred toys and states of mind when you have G-spot orgasms will be ever-changing, so don't think that you need to fit into any particular mindset to check this all out, enjoy it, or even have it be something significant for you. And if G-spot play doesn't turn out to be for you, it doesn't mean that you aren't enlightened or in touch with your sexuality (or spirituality) as a woman. You will be, more than ever, even if you think the result sucks and you hate it. But chances are good that won't be the case.

Myths

In my years as a sex educator, porn reviewer and online sex culture critic, I have found that no area of the human body has generated as many crazy, often hurtful and shameful myths about it as the G-spot. Maybe the ass rivals it in stigma, lame rumors and uneducated opinion-based judgments, but many people—all of whom claim they are absolutely right—make a mind-boggling array of statements about the G-spot and female ejaculation.

Sadly, these people often cite questionable websites, or medical papers on incontinence to back up their opinions, making it all too easy to get sucked into thinking that what they say is right—and making lots of us girls feel defective when it comes to the G-spot. Here are a few of the most ridiculous and hurtful myths:

You might not have a G-spot.
Duh! Read What the G-Spot Is in the earlier section.

Every woman likes G-spot stimulation.
This myth comes from a combination of aggressive marketing of G-spot toys, books and videos, and the enthusiasm of G-spot-happy cult worshippers who forget that it's not for everyone. I'm not going to tell you that you'll like it; G-spot sensations are unlike any other kind of sexual stimulation. But many women say that G-spot stimulation, because the feelings typically center on or around the urethra, where urine leaves the body, makes them feel like they have to pee, or it reminds them of the sensation of having to urinate. Some women may find the feeling uncomfortable for a variety of reasons. And that's okay—maybe you just know you prefer clitoral or anal stimulation to orgasm. Nothing's broken if you don't like G-spot stimulation.

There's only one right way to touch it.

There are certainly some ways to stimulate your G-spot that for some women seem to work better than others—for instance, G-spot stimulation usually requires a firm touch—but like anything related to sex and orgasm, there is no one "right" or "normal" way to make yourself feel good. Like the idea that the G-spot is some kind of magic-button instant orgasm delivery system, other information about the G-spot has been compressed into narrowly defined bite-sized chunks of advice, all too often making us think (or sometimes outright telling us) that it's like making a delicate pastry or soufflé, where one wrong step or ingredient will spoil the crust, sink the soufflé, or make your dough fall apart. It's just not so. There are lots of ways to play with your G-spot, and I'll explain a whole lot of them in the following chapters so you can mix and match and find the right combination for you.

G-spot stimulation makes you incontinent.

This is a hurtful myth based on the shaming lie that female ejaculatory fluid is urine (it's not). The people who espouse this lie will also have you believe that G-spot stimulation will make it hard for you to hold your pee if you even come near your G-spot with a vibrator. In fact, it's the opposite that's true:

G-spot stimulation brings blood and muscular activity to the entire area, strengthening it just as you
would a muscle at the gym, making your control more
precise and your orgasms more powerful as you "flex"
this orgasm technique. See chapter 5, Wet Spots:
Ejaculation.

Any other orgasms are inferior to a G-spot orgasm.
There's no such thing as a bad orgasm. Mostly it's
people who love G-spot play who make this claim;
the problem is that they tend to make us think that
our incredible clitoral, vaginal or anal orgasms
somehow don't stack up. Of course they do. But G-
spot orgasms *are* pretty intense; it's just that the
women for whom G-spot orgasms are best tend to
forget that other women might prefer clitoral
orgasms. Or they may enjoy a variety of ways of
reaching orgasm, with G-spot orgasms being only
one of them. Orgasms of all kinds can range in
intensity and pleasure from blah to "Holy shit—I
think my head just exploded, is my head still
attached?" When you find a great way to come and
it's reliably intense and wonderful, it's easy to think
that's the ultimate. But it doesn't mean that other
orgasms are inferior, or that your experiences won't
change over time. So don't ever think you're less
than, or missing out if you don't have a G-spot

orgasm, or you find that you don't particularly like
G-spot stimulation.

Why It's a G

The G-spot is named after Dr. Ernest Grafenberg, a
German gynecologist and researcher who primarily
focused his studies on contraceptive research in the
1920s and '30s; unfortunately his work in the field
of contraception became illegal in Nazi Germany, and
the doctor spent time in prison before eventually
being smuggled out of the country to safety. American
sexologists, most notably Margaret Sanger of New
York, negotiated his release.* In the United States
he continued his contraception research, eventually
publishing a paper about the role of the urethra in
female orgasm in 1950. It was this groundbreaking
paper that led to more research and numerous studies about the urethra and orgasm, and female
ejaculation—as well as leading Dr. Beverly Whipple
and her colleague Dr. John D. Perry to name the area
after Grafenberg.

---

* This information comes from "Ernest Grafenberg: From Berlin to New York,"
  a paper presented by Beverly Whipple at the 5th Congress of the European
  Federation of Sexology in Berlin, June 29–July 2, 2000, and later published
  in the *Scandinavian Journal of Sexology*, Vol.3, No.2: August 2000, pp. 43–49.
  http://www2.hu-Berlin.de/sexology/GESUND/ARCHIV/GRAFENBERG.HTM

Hence, the G. It's not a random letter, nor was it named by some guy who wanted to plant his name in the female body like some astronaut landing on an exotic planet and claiming it for his home country. Nope, the spot was named by a woman for a colleague who risked a lot to develop IUDs and cervical caps at a time when people were being killed for homosexuality in Germany and actually dared to talk about female orgasm when the United States was checking out the Kinsey reports and flailing about madly for smelling salts like an uptight schoolmarm who pretends that no one exists below the waist.

But now we can say, "What's up, G?" The name might not have much meaning for us by contemporary standards, but it's got some cool history. Call it what you want. Just don't forget the lube.

what's inside a girl

The first rule about G-spot stimulation is: Know everything you can about your anatomy. This chapter is an anatomy lesson, but it's not like any you've ever read before. We all know about reproduction—the what and how of baby-making and birthing in relation to our genitals. Even if we're fuzzy on a few details, most adult women have a pretty good idea about how our pussies work for conception and birth, or at least know our way around some kind of birth control. It is a universal assumption that we know all about our reproductive anatomy and know which side is up with condoms. Most of us know about sexually transmitted infections and staying safe (or managing a virus, or curing an infection).

The thing is, even if we get any type of formal education about female genitals, none of it has anything
to do with pleasure—how to make ourselves feel
oh-so-good. Chances are, if you got any information about your pussy in school, it was in the form
of illustrated internal anatomical drawings and
estimates on how much you bleed a month and for
how long—then a lesson on how pregnancy occurs.
That's a great bit of info—but it's missing the critical fact that this part of our bodies feels good (which
I think should come first, to explain why we'd stimulate our genitals in the first place). As for critical
life skills for smart girls, learning how to be sexually self-reliant and understanding how our
pleasure systems work should be at the top of the
survival list.

While this chapter is focused on what's inside
our pussies, refreshingly, it has nothing to do with
reproduction. Welcome to the world of pleasure-
based female genital anatomy—specifically, your
G-spot and all of the interconnected systems it
works in tandem with, your clitoris and all of the
tissues inside your pelvis. Yes it's *that* connected,
and no, they never told you that in school. The more
you know about your pleasure anatomy, the more
pleasure you can wring out of your luscious little
spot.

Anatomy

Look down. What do you see? The pubic mound (or *mons veneris*, mound of Venus). This is the area over the pubic bone, usually covered with hair, and it tapers down and between your thighs, where the inner thighs meet the torso, and splits neatly around the vaginal opening.

Spread your legs and you'll see the outer lips, or outer labia, of your vagina; these are fleshy and the skin is soft and sensitive, though somewhat similar to the skin on the rest of your body (the delicate parts, at least). Unlike the smooth, hairless inner lips to be found just inside, the outer labia reside on the outside of the body and are often covered with a continuation of your pubic mound's hair. The outer lips can be compared to the male scrotum—they are similar enough in structure and evolutionary origin, and both are formed from the same tissue in utero—but obviously they differ in function. The outer labia's appearance ranges from fleshy (puffy, covering the clitoris and vaginal opening) to thin (flat, revealing the clitoral hood).

Just inside the outer lips you'll see a hairless second set of lips that surround the vaginal opening. The inner labia are definitely more liplike in color, texture and shape than the outer set, and as with every other body part, no two individuals' are alike.

The inner labia come in countless colors; beige-orange hues, pinks and even purples, wine shades, or deep brown. The color may deepen after a woman has a child, and they can even be different colors from one another. Your inner lips might be petite and flat, curled inward, fluted, or flared, or they may protrude past the pubic hair—or, often, one might protrude more than the other. Textures range from smooth to glassy, translucent to deeply crinkled.

The outer edges of each inner lip meet toward the anus at the perineum (the wall separating the vaginal canal and anus), and also up top, toward the pubic bone, where they join to create the clitoral hood— the flesh covering your clitoris. It's interesting to note that some women report enjoying stimulation of the inner lips more than clitoral stimulation. Your inner labia are chock-full of sensitive nerve endings.

The top corner of the inner lips comes to an *A* shape underneath a tight jacket of flesh covering the protruding tip of the clitoris, or glans. Though this word sounds like *gland*, the slightly bulbous, spade-shaped head of the clitoral shaft isn't a gland at all. *Glans* means "a small, round mass or body" and "tissue that can swell or harden."

The shaft of the clitoris is the portion that runs from the bottom of the inner labia's A-frame housing to the tip of the glans (the bottom edges of the *A* being

the lower boundary of the visible portion of the clitoris). The entire covering, the clitoris's whole
house, is called the hood. This protective covering
or hood encompasses the shaft in its A shape and can
range in appearance from fleshy and fat to pulled tight
and flat. Sometimes all it takes to expose the tip of
your glans is pulling back the hood; or, it may not
become visible until you're aroused. The glans is

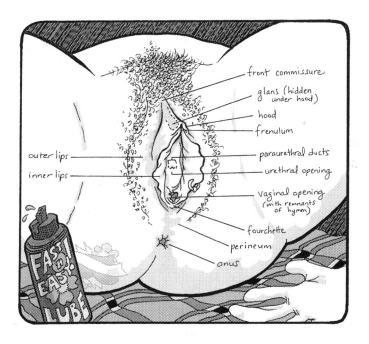

Illustration 1: External Female Anatomy

nestled in the hood and comes in many sizes, from the size of a pen tip to larger than a fingertip.

Your clitoris has eight thousand nerve endings, all concentrated in that one little spot. It contains more nerve endings than any other part of the human body, male or female, more than the fingertips, tongue or anus—and twice as many as the entire penis.

Your clitoris has but one job: your pleasure. Its function is hotly contested by evolutionary theorists (who dare to speak its name), and ignored altogether by most medical and religious institutions who can't seem to find a use for it. That's okay—*we* can figure out what to do with it. Its impracticality is ludicrous, laughable and luscious. For most women, stimula- tion of the clitoris is essential to orgasm. The clitoris is often referred to as the "powerhouse of orgasm," and though it delivers pleasure pure of purpose, touching it directly in an unaroused state can feel painful—sometimes even if you're aroused it's just too much sensation to bear. Luckily, the clitoris is shrouded by the clitoral hood, that little nub anal- ogous to the foreskin on a man, though far more sensitive. It both protects the clitoris and diffuses the sensations of touching it; even so, some women find that having their clitoral hood touched is too intense and prefer indirect clitoral stimulation, or stimulation by way of the vulva.

The area of the clitoris is far larger than described
in conventional anatomy texts and most sex guides.
The external tip, or glans, is really the tip of the
iceberg—the glans begins at the tip of the shaft and
continues under the surface to where the other end
connects to the suspensory ligament at the pubic
mound. You can feel this connection between your
clit and the pubic bone by rolling your finger across
the area; it feels somewhat like a soda straw (and
feels firmer when you're aroused). The shaft, like the
glans, is very sensitive and responds pleasurably to
stimulation. At the shaft's connection to your pubic
bone, the clitoris runs underneath both sides of your
vulva alongside the vaginal opening in a wishbone

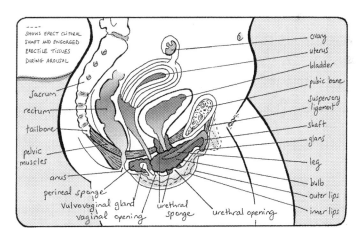

Illustration 2. Internal Female Anatomy

shape, forming two legs, or crura, and extends all the way to your perineum.

The internal area occupied by the clitoris and crura is actually a complex clitoral system, wrapped in erectile tissue—just like the stuff that fills with blood during arousal to make a penis hard. The connecting nerves, tissues, muscles, and ligaments all react and engage with one another during your arousal cycle. And guess what? Your G-spot has the princess seat right in the middle of all this. The clitoral area underneath the inner and outer lips, the ring around the urethra (where urine leaves the body), and the wall of the perineum all contain erectile tissues that fill with blood and swell upon arousal—sometimes noticeably, sometimes not. Several layers of muscles line the pelvic floor, connecting the clitoris to these erectile tissues. An oval-shaped muscle of erectile tissue surrounds the inner lips and clitoris, where the vagina and G-spot pass through it, and connects to another oval that surrounds the anal sphincter muscle, encircling the anus.

Spot Mapping

The second rule of G-spot play is: Everyone's different. From thumbprints to eyes, these may be things we all have but how they appear, feel and express their permutations is always going to differ from girl to girl. Sexual pleasure, and the G-spot, are not exceptions. How your G-spot looks and feels to touch will be as unique to you as your fingerprints and the makeup of your genital anatomy.

But some generalities apply, such as urethral anatomy—that's G-spot anatomy in case you skipped the previous sections. Both women and men have an identical ring of spongy erectile tissue surrounding the urethra (where urine leaves the body). It is an essential part of the clitoral system and your entire orgasmic network, and even when you simply jack off through clitoral stimulation, your G-spot participates in the orgasm (but more on that in the next chapter). Located inside the vagina, the urethra is a tube that's roughly two inches long, running from the bladder to the urethral opening on your vaginal wall. This ring of urethral tissue is the outer area that shows you where your G-spot is.

The urethral sponge is located on the front wall of the vagina, toward the belly button; if you're lying on your back, it's the "top" of the vaginal wall. Starting from the vaginal opening, it's roughly one or two inches inside. The outer area is the marker to let you know where the G-spot actually begins, because there's a lot more of it beneath the surface. In addition to the two-inch long urethral canal

leading to the bladder, there is a whole lot more
tissue surrounding the urethral opening (and
sponge) that makes up the entirety of the G-spot,
and it all responds to G-spot stimulation; to enjoy
your spot and come, you'll be touching not just the
urethral opening but the area surrounding it as well.

The spongy tissues that surround your urethra and
comprise your G-spot are a complex bundle of—joy!
Along with the erectile tissue, you've also got the
nerve-rich urethra itself and about forty super-tiny
glands and ducts (called paraurethral glands, or
Skene's glands) that respond to arousal and pleasure.
Sometimes, and in some women, stimulation of the
G-spot to orgasm can result in an expulsion of fluid
from the urethral sponge. This is female ejaculation
(detailed in chapter 5, Wet Spots: Ejaculation), and
the paraurethral glands and ducts have the starring
role in that particular wet, wonderful show. The purpose of the urethra is certainly to have a river run
through it, but everything else prefers to play by the
same rules as your clitoris: just for fun, thanks.

How to Get There from Here

Want to feel it? One way is to stop a stream of urine,
mid-flow. Doing this, you're flexing your PC muscles (the sling of pelvic muscles that engage during

orgasm) and putting acute pressure on your G-spot to *flex*. Another way to investigate the G-spot is with your fingers—putting a finger or two just inside your vagina and stroking the front wall. You'll have to curl your hand around a bit to get your fingertip to stroke the front wall, so sitting down on a stool or hard chair might make it easier for you to spread your legs, push your pelvis forward, and feel. I highly recommend using a water- or silicone-based lubricant in your explorations, as different surfaces are easier to detect under slick fingertips. I recommend a variety of excellent lubricants for G-spot exploration in chapter 3, Turn It On, Turn It Up.

What you're feeling for is a soft bump or slight change in the surface of your vaginal wall. If you touch yourself just inside your vagina, you'll notice that the surface near the opening is slightly furrowed with subtle ridges, and a bit more so in the area where you'll be concentrating your search for the urethral opening. It's interesting to note that this ridgy outer area of the vaginal canal (about the inner third) is more sensitive to touch, vibration and more subtle textures and shapes than the smooth-walled inner part (the inner two thirds), which cares less about vibration and responds pleasurably to sensations like fullness, rhythm and thrusting. If you're feeling like exploring, touch and press all around your urethral opening while squeezing your vaginal muscles and see if you can feel what's beneath the surface.

If you're unaroused, the urethral sponge is relaxed and might be difficult to feel. But during arousal, your sponge swells and hardens, and it becomes more obvious to touch. Touching it in an unaroused state might feel strange, like you have to pee a bit, or it might be too sensitive to touch—or it might feel good. It might even feel *really* good. You may find that touching it turns you on a little, and that once your G-spot is firm with arousal, massage and vibration are delightful. Just try a simple touch once, and see how your body responds.

Exploring your G-spot with touch to see what it feels like under your fingertips while it is in an aroused state is a whole different experience (and a highly recommended one, I might add). When you're turned on, not only might it feel good to touch but, as I've indicated above, it'll be easier to locate the spot because when you're aroused, the entire area swells and the urethral sponge becomes firm— sometimes very firm—to the touch. One great way to do this is to arouse yourself in a familiar way, maybe using your favorite masturbation technique. Do whatever you feel like to get yourself in the mood and horny; use a favored sex toy or fantasy; watch porn, or read some hot erotica. Once you can't keep your hands out of your panties any longer, play with yourself and slip a finger inside to explore your vaginal opening—a fact-finding mission. But don't forget to keep yourself turned on while you do it (for the best results, of course).

What the G-Spot Looks Like

Maybe you're the kind of smart girl who wants to see the proof—or who just wants to know what all of her excellent girl parts look like. Whether you're the girl who has to see the photographic proof that Pamela Anderson really did get a new boob job, or the kind of girl that takes apart the alarm clock to see how it works, there's only one way to satisfy your curiosity (and learn more about yourself): take a look.

For this adventure, you'll need a hand mirror—you could try and position yourself in front of a full-length mirror while sitting in a chair, but to really see the tiny urethral opening you'll need to get up close with the mirror and angle it. It's a two-handed operation, and one that also requires a good light source. See if you can get a reading lamp or goose-necked office light for a well-lit exam. If not, be sure to sit facing a light source and you should be able to see everything just fine.

Sit on the edge of a chair or your bathtub, spread your legs, and roll your torso forward slightly, tilting your pelvis and pulling your ass cheeks back from your pussy using the chair as leverage. With one hand, split your fingers along each side of your vaginal opening and spread your inner and outer labia open, lifting upward.

If you take a look at it when you're turned on, you'll probably see a whole different shape and size than if you're unaroused. When you get turned on, the acorn shape swells and the area around it puffs out—sometimes only a little, sometimes quite a bit. You may also notice the area has changed color, deepening in tone; some areas may look more highlighted than others. In some women the soft urethral sponge retreats in an unaroused state, making you have to hunt around for it a bit. When unaroused, your G-spot area is going to look somewhat like an acorn with tiny folds of flesh around it—and you may even be able to see a little opening. Yay! That's it!

turn it on,
turn it up

So now that you no longer need to use Google Maps to find your G-spot, what are you going to do with it? Have a really great time, that's what. Figuring out where to aim when you're stimulating your G-spot is half of the equation; the other half is figuring out how. Do you think you'll like fingers, a vibrator, a glass wand, a penis, or a strap-on? Will you want it firm right off the bat, or a deep massage followed by thrusts, or is size your favorite way to come *à la G*?

Even though it sounds like there might be a lot of options, figuring out what you like for your G-spot sessions is really the easy part—just do what feels good. But understanding your arousal cycle might give you even more insight into ramping up your sex life in general—and not just for G-spot play, though it'll certainly make the G-spot a much easier little sex toy to operate, control and utilize to its fullest potential. After that, it's just a matter of trying different techniques to see what works best and when it works for you, and a few technical details about G-spot play, in addition to seeing what kind of accessories might make your sessions hotter than ever.

Your Arousal Cycle

Some really cool stuff happens to your entire body when you're turned on. When you become sexually aroused, your senses and genitals shift from their ordinary everyday mode into a much more surreal realm. In this state, mentally, physically and sometimes emotionally, pleasure is the guiding force behind all of your actions and the chief driver of your thoughts; your entire body begins to respond physically to the chemicals and hormones flooding from brain to bloodstream. Without you even thinking about it, blood rushes to your pelvis, filling the erectile tissues, and all of the nerve cells in your genitals become active, awake. Believe it or not, your breasts increase slightly in size. Stimulation of the nipples might make everything feel that much more intense, as nipple stimulation causes production of the hormone oxytocin, which is produced during sexual stimulation and causes tingling sensations in the genitals. The skin on various parts of your body becomes hypersensitive, and your nipples and genitals flush and deepen in color.

Because the erectile tissue in your genitals is analogous to the erectile tissue in the penis, it also swells when aroused. You might see a noticeable change in the landscape of your pussy (or not); the outer lips might puff, the clit may grow larger and firmer, and if you peek at your G-spot you'll likely see it has become bigger, fatter. What's cool about our erectile tissue is that unlike that in a male's penis, there are no muscles that compress the blood flow to retain stiffness—we don't have a shutoff valve to keep the erection and then release blood after ejaculation— and perhaps that is where we women get our capacity for multiple orgasms. It's a constant ebb and flow, until we're done. Yay for us!

The clit really gets busy when we get turned on. During arousal, clitoral erection pushes the glans forward, and it may poke out from under the hood. Underneath the surface, the clitoral legs and surrounding erectile tissue stiffen, elongate, and swell, expanding both inner and outer labia. This all colludes to put a divine pressure on the G-spot.

Inside your inner labia lips there are two tiny ducts connected to two tiny glands called the vulvovaginal glands, which produce a few drops of thick fluid during arousal. This contributes to, but does not compose entirely, vaginal lubrication during the sexual response cycle. Pressure from dilated clitoral blood vessels inside the vagina during arousal forces clear fluid through the walls of the vagina, which is where the majority of vaginal lubrication comes from. However, lubrication is not a reliable means by which to measure arousal. You can be lubricated yet unaroused, and you can just as easily be chomping at the bit for sex and have a dry vulva. Lubrication varies depending on mood, stress, where you are in your menstrual cycle, whether you've experienced menopause, medications and antihistamines you've taken, and any number of other factors.

As your arousal heightens, all the muscles and ligaments begin to contract, creating a delightful tension. The suspensory ligament connected to your clit shortens and pulls the glans inward toward the pubic bone, and it may remains beneath the hood until orgasm. The end of the round ligament tugs on the inner lips at one end and the uterus on the other, creating more pleasure and involving the uterus in the orgasmic process. It's like an awesome system of weights, pulleys and muscular communication, and the G-spot is right in the middle of all this action.

As you get closer to orgasm, your pelvic muscle tension is building and your body is working in concert with your pussy as the conductor: the clitoral tissues and perineum are hypersensitive, as is the skin on your face, neck, abdomen, buttocks, hands and feet. Blood pressure and heart rate are increased. Your entire body is awash in sexual chemicals, and this strong chemical and hormonal cocktail is making even your vision more vivid and hyperreal, all while demanding the inevitable release. When you go over the edge and come, your pelvic muscular tension explodes in a series of short, rhythmic contractions. The walls of the vagina, and all the muscles on the pelvic floor, contract strongly and rhythmically, causing intense pleasure. Your vagina squeezes, your clit pulses, your anus pushes and your G-spot constricts itself in an orgasmic embrace—sometimes pushing out fluid from the sponge and paraurethral glands. This is orgasm, and you have a buffet of styles to choose from, in addition to being able to come back for seconds, thirds or even more.

How to Stimulate Your Spot

The very first order of business when you want to play pleasurably with your G-spot is to begin from an aroused state. This is for a number of good reasons.

One is that if you're new to G-spot stimulation, it will really help your attitude going into trying a new, unfamiliar and possibly daunting sexual activity, and arousal will make the road over new physical sensations a lot smoother to travel. Another good reason is that many women who enjoy G-spot play only like to do it once they're rarin' to go; starting out with G-spot stimulation alone leaves many women cold. And finally, some women really like G-spot stimulation only after they've had an orgasm.

Before you start, go pee. Then get yourself turned on, or keep any potential G-spot toys at the ready for when you do feel extra horny and want to experiment with your spot. Use any means you prefer for getting turned on; porn, fantasy, heavy petting with a lover, your favorite toys—whatever you like the most at that moment. Masturbate and bring yourself to a point of orgasmic urgency, where you really want to take yourself to the next level and orgasm. Put a vibrator on your clit, and play with it there for a while. Then reach for the lube, and start your G-spot stimulation.

G-spot stimulation requires firm pressure; it takes a strong touch or a solid sex toy, and you'll find that it feels best when you really press toward the front of your body. You may be able to touch the urethral opening, but the entirety of the G-spot is behind that, within the vaginal wall. That's what you're aiming for. Start with a little pressure at first and try out pulses, up and down strokes, side-to-side motions, or even moving in lazy circles over the area that feels best. Pay attention to how different techniques feel as you try them out, and take note of the ones you like the most. Go at your own pace with adding or lifting pressure on your G-spot as you take in all of the physical data your body is sending you about what you're doing.

How It Feels

If this is the first time you've tried this, it's going to feel…intense. New. It won't feel like anything else you've ever tried, sensation-wise, for sex. The first thing you'll notice is that you're pressing on your bladder area from an unfamiliar angle, which is a big reason I recommend that you pee before you start. Many women report that the pressure required to adequately massage their G-spots makes them feel like they have to urinate. This is typical—though it's not the case for everyone. Some girls find that the urge to pee is just too much of the wrong kind of signal to be getting when they're masturbating, and decide that G-spot play isn't for them. And that's okay! Even if you decide that this isn't for you,

you've explored it adequately and now you know the role your G-spot plays in orgasm and sex, even if you decline to utilize it through direct stimulation.

However, a good number of women find that this urgency to urinate soon passes—or they "push through it"—and many see this sensation as the gateway to the next level of G-spot pleasure. The general opinion is that there is a biting urge to pee for several strokes, and then the arousal moves into a deeper, more intense sense of pleasurable stimulation that is a full-body sensation, as opposed to clitoral stimulation that feels like it's on the outside, or anal stimulation that tends to feel like it's in the back of the body. G-spot pleasure resides right in the middle of your body, radiating from the core. This is certain: a G-spot orgasm is *very* different from a clitoral orgasm.

The feeling will begin to build, and you'll find that you want stronger, harder strokes. In fact, it may amaze you to find out how hard you can (and how hard you want to) press against your vagina's anterior wall. Don't worry—you can't hurt anything as long as you have a nice, smooth toy (or smooth fingers) and plenty of lube. The vagina is incredible; during arousal it can stretch to many times its natural size and after you're done it shrinks right back. We're made to do that, and in fact when we push our pussies to their limits we make them stronger, heartier and more powerful by exercising the remarkable muscles and ligaments that come into play and the full range of our sexual response. It is just like exercise; the more we do it, the healthier and more resilient we become.

Your G-spot will tell you what to do; press harder, stroke faster; shorter thrusts, more fullness, or even more lube or vibration (if you're using a vibrator). It could be that what you're using isn't enough in terms of fullness, which is why a significant number of G-spot aficionados require more than two fingers—a fist will do nicely for them, thank you very much, and look out when she comes.

Sex Toys

Using fingers to stimulate your G-spot is a wonderful way to go—whether they're yours or your lover's. Even better, a set of gifted fingers inside a latex (or nonlatex) glove can heighten the pleasure with the increased smoothness and firmer touch the gloves provide. However, most women really enjoy the results they get with sex toys—hard dildos made of silicone, glass, acrylic, hard plastic, wood or stone; and firm vibrators with a nice curve and smooth tip. Plus, hands and fingers get tired, mobility might be an issue, and variation is the spice of a smart girl's life—indeed.

There are about a zillion toys marketed for G-spot use, and some of them are perfectly awesome for your spot; others are obviously just regular toys with the word *G-spot* slapped on the package, while the toy itself will prove useless for your G-spot needs. You can tell the difference between good and lame G-spot toys by following some pretty basic criteria.

G-spot toys need to be firm, slightly curved, and should look like they can reach up like a finger in a "come here" gesture. If you're not sure about choosing a G-spot toy in a cold shopping experiment, many women-run sex toy shops sell G-spot exploration kits specifically aimed at beginners; these are a great starter item. Typically, the main toy in these kits is a hard plastic or firm jelly rubber curved vibrator, as lots of women find that vibration makes G-spot exploration more fun to start playing with.

Toys in hard materials (like silicone, hard plastic, glass, metal or stone) are well-suited for G-spot play for obvious reasons, and they have the added bonus of being nonporous, meaning they're easy to clean and don't retain bacteria in the tiny pockets or pores in the surface. This means that when you clean one of these toys, it's completely clean and doesn't have the potential to carry STDs or bacteria that can infect (or reinfect) the user. Plastic, glass and Pyrex, metal, and stone sex toys can have their surfaces rendered sterile by washing with unscented antibacterial soap (like Hibiclens) or a solution of 1:10 bleach and water (1:10 rubbing alcohol and water is a fine alternative).

Silicone is an excellent choice for your G-spot toys, as it is completely nonporous, retains heat and transmits vibration wonderfully, and is easy to sterilize. The thing is, not all silicone toys are the same when it comes to firmness; some are floppy and soft while others are hard enough to get the job done nicely. Make sure the silicone toy you buy is hard—read, ask questions and see if you can handle the toy in a store before you pay the extra money for one of these high-quality toys. Silicone toys can be boiled for up to five minutes or run in the top rack of the dishwasher for complete sterilization, which is especially awesome for anal toys. Some silicone toys react badly to silicone lubricants, so it's best to use water-based lubes with your silicone toys.

Most sex toys are made of a material usually referred to as jelly rubber, though you'll also see variations like jel-lee, latex jelly, or derivatives like glow-in-the-dark and "realistic" materials such as softskin, Cyberskin, or Futurotic. Jelly rubber toys are very colorful, clear (though not always), shiny, and visually appealing. They're fashioned out of the ultimate "mystery material," mass-produced mostly in Chinese chemical factories with so many mixtures and versions of the material that it's difficult to pin down a set of manufacturer's ingredients. What *is* known, however, is that these materials contain latex, give off a highly chemical smell, leach oils and can leave spots on fabrics and wood, and have a surface that breaks down over time.

Some jelly rubber toys will be great for your G-spot fun; they're inexpensive, often come in shapes and options you can't find in higher-quality materials and can last a long time despite their cheap manufacturing process. Take my advice to keep the surface totally clean: always use these toys with a condom over them. Even if you have no reaction to jelly rubber, and most people don't, remember to keep the toy scrupulously clean. Wash such toys with unscented antibacterial soap (like Hibiclens) or a solution of 1:10 bleach and water (alcohol and water also works fine). Waterproof G-spot toys are wonderful in this regard, as they can be completely submerged during cleaning. Consider porous toys disposable. Keep an eye on the surface; once it becomes dull, it's starting to break down and you can never be sure you're getting it clean; so be safe— toss it out and get a new one.

Lube

Lube is definitely on the must-have list for G-spot play—and even if you've never tried lube, you won't believe what you've been missing. Lubricant makes everything wonderfully slippery and heightens sensations, while reducing skin "drag" that some women find distracting or even unpleasant during G-spot stimulation.

Lube comes in a mind-boggling selection: there are more thicknesses, consistencies, flavors, and styles than can be listed here. Finding the lube that's right for you will be a matter of personal preference, though some women like different lubes for certain activities, or even as different moods strike. Some lubes closely mimic natural vaginal lubrication (like Liquid Silk); others will be thick and gel-like with lots of staying power and can make inserting big objects easier (like Slippery Stuff Gel). Or, you may find that sometimes you prefer long-lasting silicone-based lubes like Eros Silicone for their ability to mimic oil without the unwanted difficulty of cleaning oils out of the vagina (silicone is water-soluble).

Water-based lubes are at the top of the most-recommended list as they have a lot of convenient features: they clean up easily with water and are easily flushed from your vaginal ecosystem. Oils of any kind are difficult to get out of the vagina, and also break down latex, foiling any safer-sex plans you might have. Some water-based lubes have sugars (also labeled glycerin, glycerol, and natural flavor) that are very irritating to many women; since sugar feeds yeast, these can lead to yeast infections. Read the ingredients list before you purchase your lube, and know that unwanted colorings and flavors can have similar undesirable effects. Water-based lubes (including silicone) are safe to use with condoms and safer-sex gear.

Please do avoid vaginal "shrink creams" sold in porn and adult "novelty" stores, which claim to make the vagina smaller or tighter. The key ingredient in these creams is alum (aluminum chloride, an aluminum compound). They absorb water from the outer layer of the skin; as more water is absorbed, the cells begin to swell, closing the ducts through which water would normally flow. No study has been done on the effect of these creams on the cervix or urethra, which is what they eventually end up getting rubbed on during penetration, but I'll wager it's not good.

Good to Be Wrong

ALISON TYLER

Caroline tells me that she's never masturbated. Not ever. Not even during the times when she's been single.

"Never?" I ask, in disbelief.

"Never."

I picture her years ago in her twin bed, alone, sleeping on her hands to keep from sliding them between her legs, wearing thick fleecy mittens when the urge gets really bad.

"But why not?"

She claims that whenever she has needed to come, she's always had sex with a willing partner. In fact, she acts positively insulted by the suggestion she could ever have had any trouble finding someone who wanted to take her on—don't I think she's pretty enough to attract a lover?

Of course, I do. She's stunning, slim and dark with large green eyes. She's so fucking pretty that I can't imagine she wouldn't turn herself on if she looked in a mirror. But pretty has nothing to do with this. With the urges, with the needs. I come at least every day, whether I'm with a partner, or solo. Why wouldn't she share the same type of yearnings?

"I just wouldn't stoop to using my fingers," she

explains smugly, shaking her head when I question her about a dildo, or the high-pressure massager in a shower.

Stoop? I wonder. *Who's stooping?*

I enjoy pleasuring myself, and I see nothing wrong with it, even if there is a willing partner nearby. God, *especially* when there's a willing partner nearby. I have always gotten excited when playing with myself for an audience, and I have relished watching my lovers do the same. You can learn a lot when you watch. This is probably why I relish videotaping so much. Playing back the tapes, when there is time to critique a performance, has turned me into the caring, careful lover that I am today.

"Caring," Caroline sneers. "If you were so caring, you wouldn't be pushing me to do that!"

I sigh. She just doesn't understand.

Caroline claims that the concept of masturbating feels dirty to her.

"How so?" I wonder.

"You know," she says, flushing. "Just the thought of sliding my fingertips—"

"Where?" I insist, already envisioning those well-manicured nails sliding between her pale, pink pussy lips and skimming against her clit.

"You know!" she demands. "It feels dirty."

Shit, I get hot just imagining this sultry vision, thinking about her strumming herself or me doing the actions for her. She's got such a pretty pussy. Her cunt deserves to be well-loved, well taken care of.

"Dirty," she whispers to me, in a way that only works to arouse me more.

Dirty can be good, I want to tell her. *Dirty can be fun... so much fucking fun.*

Yet I can tell she does not share my view of the word. So I try to see the situation her way. And I fail. *What's* dirty? I like the way my juices feel on my fingers. I like the way I smell, the way the nectar of my sex tastes when I lick the tips of my fingers clean afterward. I like the feeling when I've already come once, and then work myself in a different way entirely, curling my fingers up into my pussy, searching out my G-spot, going slowly and teasing that soft smooth area...knowing what unbelievable pleasures await.

We don't have this conversation often. I don't beat her up with the concept every day. But with my warped and twisted mind, I finally reach the point where all I can think of is Caroline playing with herself. This becomes my number-one masturbation fantasy: watching *her* masturbate. I try my best to catch her in the act. I sneak into the bathroom when she's showering, only to find her (drumroll, please)

showering. I stay up late, pretending to sleep, waiting to see if the bed will shake with her silent
orgasms. I deny her sex, hoping that this will drive
her to make herself come.

Doesn't work. She's like a camel, with a vast ability to store her sexual thirst.

Ultimately, I confess to her. I tell her that it would
make me very happy to see her bring herself to climax.
I feel bad pushing her, and I apologize for coming
on so strong. But, I say, I can't fucking help it. She's
driving me out of my head.

She looks at me for a long time. Then she sighs
and settles back on our bed with her slim legs apart,
and she slides her hand beneath the waistband of her
pink floral skirt. She says, "If this is so important to
you—" and I nod like a maniac, like a psycho, foam-
ing at the mouth, and I say, "Yeah, yeah, it's really
important." I hear the way I sound, but I can't keep
the excitement out of my voice.

I can tell right off that she doesn't seem to know
how to start. She fumbles with her white cotton
panties, then squints as if she's hurt herself.

"Take off your clothes," I suggest. "That might
make things easier."

She shrugs, as if she's got nothing to lose, and she
takes off her skirt and her panties, then pulls her tight
pink tank top over her head and lies back down again.

I'm watching her as if she's behind a glass partition at a sex club. I'm watching like some lecherous leering Tom with a pocketful of twenties. I cannot contain myself. I say in a husky voice, "That's my girl. Now, spread your legs wider and stroke yourself gently."

She gives me a withering stare. I shut up. And watch.

She places her fingers on her outer lips and makes small circles over her entire delta of Venus. She does this for a while before shrugging and telling me it's not working. Caroline says the words as if this is what she expected.

"I can't come like this," she explains.

"Maybe you need a toy," I suggest, but the thought makes her frown.

"Please," I try, offering her up a glass dildo, one with a bend at the end, perfect for reaching a G-spot. "But wait," I tell her, thrilled with my own brain wave. "Let me get you ready first...." And then I'm between her legs, licking her, touching her. I am so hungry for her. Caroline has no problem with this situation. She loves when I eat her out. Now, she spreads her thighs willingly, she even uses her fingers to part her pussy lips so that I can get in deep. I press my mouth against her, my tongue cradling her clit, lapping at her. And the whole time I'm fucking her with my tongue, I'm imagining her touching herself. That desire does not wane in the slightest.

I want her to show me, and yet, and yet, I'm so damn hot. I drink from her sweet font until her hips beat on the smooth satin comforter, until the first climax shatters her world, and then reluctantly, oh so reluctantly, I pull away.

"What do you want now?" Caroline asks, confused. "You saw me come."

"I've seen you come before," I remind her. "I want to see you make yourself come." I'm offering her the toy once more. I'm holding it out with shaky, sweaty fingers.

Come on, girl, I'm thinking. *Show me. Please, show me.*

She swallows hard as she takes the dildo from my fingers. It's a beautiful one, curved glass, chilly to the touch. A gift from me to her on Valentine's Day that has gone unused, unthought of, languishing in her panty drawer. She closes her eyes and leans back on the bed and begins to tickle her clit with the tip. I'm dying. She looks so pretty, and so different, sort of lost in the moment, letting herself go. Caroline never really lets go.

I steady myself and sit on my hands to keep from touching her, unconsciously mimicking the posture I've imagined her in. Where are the mittens on my fingers? I need cuffs to keep my hands under control.

I watch as she slides the toy into her pussy. A few

inches of it disappear. I lick my lips, trying to memorize every second, sure that this is a onetime show. She's not going to do this again for me, no matter how much I beg.

"Push it all the way in," I tell her.

Caroline squints, then does what I say.

"And press," I continue.

"It makes me feel like I have to pee."

"You'll get over that," I assure her. "The feeling will pass."

She gives me a look, like, *What is all of this about? Why are you tormenting me this way?* And I want to remind her that I'm the Dom. That I'm the one who likes to torment her. And I also want to remind her that it's not as if I'm threatening her with pain. I've offered her only pleasure here, if she will simply obey.

Still clearly unsure, Caroline begins to rub the toy inside herself, and I can tell when she presses beyond the feeling of wetting the bed. I can see the rose-pink flush on her cheeks as the pleasure begins to build...and build. Her hand is working more forcefully now. I can tell that she's got it. That she understands.

Suddenly, she has a look on her face that she gets when I'm fucking her really good. I move even closer, between her legs, and I put one hand on her, rolling her onto her side, bringing her knees up toward her chest. She keeps using the dildo, keeps working it, and she doesn't stop or flinch when I wrap my arms around her, when I hold her tight. She just keeps her wrist going in this crazy rhythm, fucking herself.

I lean up on one arm and watch her face to see her pleasure crest. Her eyelids flutter as she starts to peak. She stares at me, whispers my name, coming, coming, fulfilling my fantasy...and then her hand stops working, rests limply between her legs. Her body is still shuddering, though, as if aftershocks of pleasure continue to work her from the inside.

I withdraw the toy for her and set the lovely wet glass dildo on the bedside table. Then I take her into my arms and call her my angel, tell her how turned on I am, how ravishing she is.

Sweetly, she turns in my arms and presses her hips forward, climbing on top of me and kissing me. "Oh, god," she says, and I grin at her. "That was so good," she says, and I realize from the look in her eyes that she *will* do it again for me. That there *will* be a repeat performance.

Sometimes it's good to be wrong.

g-spots are for sharing

We girls come stocked with so many cool sex features—like fun-to-play-with breasts, sensitive clits, and a tireless capacity for orgasm. We are hardwired to enjoy sex, and we are certainly programmed to share it. Sure it's fun to play with ourselves all day. But it's even more fun to share our pleasure zones with a playmate. Our G-spots are the ultimate in shareable pleasure parts.

Why do I think G-spot play is the ultimate in sexual shareware? Lots of reasons. Number one is that the G-spot's in an area that is often more easily accessed by a lover; as I mentioned in previous chapters, the angle and pressure many women find necessary to stimulate their spots pleasurably is often better accomplished by someone else. Another great reason, especially for G-spot newcomers, is that finding and learning about the G-spot can be both easier and more fun when you have a partner helping you figure out what you like. You can just lie back and let someone else's fingers (or more) do the walking. And sometimes the pleasure and overwhelming sensations of G-spot orgasm are so intense you may need help getting over the top—and back again. A G-spot adventure shared by two is an incredibly intimate experience.

Talk about It

Maybe you've always enjoyed G-spot play yourself and now you want to teach a lover how to maximize your spot. You might be totally new to G-spot exploration and want to ask your sweetie to try it out with you. Or you could be new to it and trying G-spot play isn't even your idea, but rather your partner's suggestion for new sexual thrills. It could be that you're the one who wants to ask your lover if she'd like to try some G-spot toys and techniques, but you aren't sure how to proceed.

The first step in each of these different situations is learning G-spot mechanics and techniques, and then talking about what you want, or what you think you might want, or what you're worried about, or what your wildest G-spot dreams are, with your lover.

This means you have to bring it up, mention it, or somehow get a conversation started about sex— G-spot play, specifically—and start to figure out what you both want to do about it.

How to Start the Conversation

If talking about sex is something that comes naturally in your relationship, then you're off to a sweet start. The next time you feel the conversation drifting toward sex, simply mention that you'd like to try something new, or that you saw some interesting sex toys for G-spot play that caught your attention, or that you read an article about G-spot stimulation and you'd like to try it—with your partner's help, of course. Next, go over the finer points of anatomy in this book; then jot down a toy, lube and safer-sex gear shopping list, and make a playdate. You can even make it into an evening filled with sensual delights: aphrodisiac nibbles, sexy music, low lighting and plenty of distraction-free time to play with getting yourselves turned on and tuned in to your (or her) G-spot.

What If You Don't Usually Talk about Sex?

What if sex talk is infrequent in your relationship, but you want to start a conversation about trying G-spot play? In this situation, you know what you want, but don't know how to get it. And there's the added stress of knowing that once you get your courage up to ask, it doesn't mean you'll be met with enthusiasm; or if you are, that your lover will be able to execute your desires in the ways you want. Opening up can be scary, and being met with shock, surprise, or distaste is even scarier. Learning how to talk about each other's desires, and gleaning a few tips for starting the conversation, are where you'll want to begin.

Talking about sex brings you closer together, period. You both get to find out each other's sexiest secret wishes, and how to make them come true. You embark on a sexual adventure that takes you into exciting new territory and far away from your old sex routines. And for your relationship, your willingness to try new things takes you both to the next level.

Fantasy Fuels G-Spot Play

Our erotic fantasies are what lead us into wanting to try new things sexually with each other. These urges and ideas can come from some of the deepest parts of ourselves—even if they often don't *feel* like they do when you want to open your mouth and talk about them. When you share your sexual ideas with each other, you're being allowed into each other's most private worlds. It's easy to feel emotionally exposed. You have to trust your partner to withhold judgment about you and why you want to change your sexual routines in the first place. Though these fears can be largely addressed by talking about it together, moving through that hard part—getting started— takes trust.

Not everyone is going to feel vulnerable and freaked out asking to try out G-spot play; some will be empowered; most will feel finally free to truly express themselves sexually; and many others are just going to enjoy having another excuse to have hot(ter) sex. Trying out new things like G-spot play can keep your relationship strong, vibrant and alive.

Ultimately it's as simple—and as nerve-wracking— as asking. First, whose idea is this? Is it your fantasy, your lover's, or both? If it's yours, all you need to do is tell your partner what you want. Trying new things in bed (or out of bed, as you please) starts with an idea and can become reality as easily as making a wish—as long as you make that wish out loud. Those readers who are introducing the G-spot to their partners as a new idea might receive a mixed reply— part curiosity, part apprehension. You may even be met with a reluctance to talk about it, while others might get an outright "no thanks." Opening yourself up and asking for something you want sexually takes courage—but it also gives you an opportunity to learn more about what your lover likes and dislikes.

If you're the one bringing it up, reverse roles for a minute: If you don't normally talk about sex in your relationship and then suddenly one of you wants to, it might seem like an upsetting surprise—at first. Your lover may wonder if you've had sexual secrets all along. But it's very likely that opening up about your desires for more sexual pleasure (together!) will give your sweetie the opportunity to tell you what's on her mind about sex, too.

Before you begin, think about how you might bring up the subject in a way that would feel safe for you. Mention an article you saw in a magazine or on the Web, a book you saw about the G-spot, or a conversation you overheard. Do you think you'd feel okay asking your partner what he or she thinks about G-spot play while cuddling?

Consider ways in which you can encourage your partner to hear you out, and ask him to suspend judgment until you can explain why this is important, and how much fun you think the two of you will both have. Let your lover know that if she tries it and doesn't like it, that's totally okay, too. Be sure to reassure him or her that you find him incredibly sexy, and that this wouldn't be happening unless you felt safe to tell her your deepest desires. Your lover needs to hear that he or she is the star of your show, whether giving or receiving G-spot play, in addition to the fact that you're ready to become closer than you've ever been before. The most important thing to think through beforehand is how you are going to make your partner feel safe when talking about it. Rehearse what you'd like to say in your mind before you actu- ally have the conversation. Think through possible scenarios, and imagine how your lover might react, so that you will be prepared to flow with whichever route the discussion might take.

For many reasons, your lover may not want to try G-spot exploration. Understanding these concerns and hesitations can be helpful in having a construc- tive discussion about it, learning how to overcome fears that might hold one of you back, and resolving what to do when one person does feels okay about it while the other doesn't. Adding any new sexual behavior to a relationship can feel like a make-or- break situation, and sometimes it is. Asking to try new styles of expressing sexual intimacy can push your relationship to higher levels, or it can bring up so many issues that it rocks the boat—sometimes a little too hard. When sex makes someone feel inse- cure, uncomfortable or unsure of your motivations, the issues can rock that person to the core. This is especially true for survivors of sexual trauma or abuse.

Take this into your considerations: sometimes our reluctances or concerns come from cultural stigma about our own body parts—our vaginas. The one thing we women do learn about our sexuality growing up is that our vaginas are dirty things, and millions of dollars go into douche and tampon commercials to prove it. Actually, the notion of female sexual organs being filthy has the theological backing of more than a few religions, and cultural roots centuries deep. And it's all very dated.

We hear jokes about fish. We get cultural messages about being gross. We see men's magazines and worry that we don't stack up in every way—no one's pussy looks like that of a *Playboy* centerfold or porn star, and that's a very good thing, since those pussies are waxed, made up, airbrushed and surgeried to within an inch of their lives. Every girl worries about whether she looks "normal," is too hairy (or not hairy enough), doesn't smell like a summer breeze; or how she might taste—and a biggie in this case, how long she might take to come.

Think about all this, and know that everything you—or your partner—may be worried about is wrong. Not having a porn star pussy is normal—and desirable. If you think you might be off in scent or taste, take a relaxing bath and avoid eating asparagus and garlic, or taking antihistamines and vitamins.

And as far as taking too long to come, stop worry-
ing and enjoy the ride—even if you don't come, you're
still having fun.

G-Spot Massage

Generally speaking, vulva massage is something that
can build and increase a woman's arousal, and can be
a terrific, languorous way to make her come. Like a regular massage, it's a very sensual form of contact and
very relaxing for the recipient. Giving her mons veneris
and vulva a massage is highly recommended, even if
it's just a stopover on your way to G-spot massage.

As a precursor, know that you should never use
oils on her vulva or in her vagina. You can give a dry
massage, but a water-based or silicone lubricant is
highly recommended. From the beginning, start
with light touches and strokes all over her torso and
abdomen, upper thighs, and hips. Cup your hand over
her vulva and hold it still for a moment; go very slowly.
Press lightly, and begin to move your hand in a circular motion. Apply a steady pressure with the palm
of your hand to her outer lips, and keep circling. Next,
move on to these massage techniques:

- With both hands, press your flattened fingertips on either side of her vulva.

- Using your thumb and forefinger on each of the outer labia, give a massaging pinch.
- Flatten both hands and stroke her outer lips, pulling up and down.
- With the same flat-hand position, press the outer labia in (toward each other), and out (away from each other).
- Use the pads of your fingertips to stroke the outer labia up and down, and massage into the furrows between the inner and outer lips.
- Flatten your palms on her thighs and massage in small circles with your thumbs, working from bottom to top. Stay to the sides of her clitoris.
- Flatten your fingers over her vaginal opening and apply pressure in small circles.
- Alternate any of these techniques with the open-hand massage you started with.

Continue your external massage techniques for a duration of about ten minutes (or until she tells you she's ready for more) before you start to move your ministrations inside the lips of her vagina. In some instances you'll just be able to "tell" when she's ready for more; she'll move closer to you, buck her hips toward your hand or make movements and noises indicating she wants more. Trust your intuition, but also don't be afraid to ask her outright if she wants more of anything you're doing. Be specific with your questions: asking if she likes it will get you a non-specific "mm-hmm," while targeted questions will get you the direction you need. Try:

- "Would you like it harder here?"
- "Is it better to the side, or in the middle?"
- "Are you ready for penetration now?"
- "More lube?"
- "Do you want the (G-spot) toy now?"

Keep massaging her clitoris and vulva with your other hand when you begin to penetrate her and massage the G-spot; look to chapter 3 for tips on how you'll want to touch her G-spot. Use your hands or a curved, firm G-spot toy, and start with slow thrusts, literally massaging the area somewhat lightly as if it were a muscle in her back. Always press forward, toward her belly button, and aim to concentrate your touch about one to two inches inside her vaginal opening. Here are a few techniques you can cycle through slowly:

- Thrust in and press the G-spot on the out-stroke.
- Try the reverse; press against the G-spot on the "in" stroke.

- Leave your fingers or the toy inside, and press for a second, then release.
- Try pressing in short pulses, or up to the length of a breath.
- Massage in a circular motion. Do this for a while and then reverse directions—or just go in one direction only.
- Try short, firm strokes for a minute, then slow ones.
- Massage the G-spot in small, tight figure-eight movements.

When things really start to heat up, pick the stroke or technique she really responds to (or tells you she likes the most) and stick with it. When you find what really works, stopping and switching is not recommended unless you want to head off her orgasm. If you want her to come, take her over the edge with the stroke that works. Chances are good you'll have to increase the pressure and speed behind whatever stroke you use to achieve orgasm. Definitely get your hand and arm muscles ready for a workout!

G-Spot vs. Strap-On

Some women really like having their G-spots stimulated during penetration, and strap-ons are a terrific way to make these women very, *very* happy. Strap-ons are ideal for G-spot fucking because a variety of dildos are available made especially for G-spot stimulation. These dildos are hard and curved, and some even have a bulbous tip designed to get just the right angle and firmness needed for a G-spot orgasm. Look for harness-compatible dildos that have a G in their name or fit all the qualifications for a G-spot toy—and especially look for dildos made by women-owned companies as they'll be designed thoughtfully for maximum G-spot pleasure. (The garden-variety porn store G-spot toys tend to be poorly designed, with little curve and often too soft to be any fun.)

Newcomers to strap-on play will want to make their first purchase an inexpensive harness made of fabric or nylon and a one-off rubber dildo in a pleasing and reasonable shape. Options for harnesses range from neoprene and nylon to glittery vinyl, rubber, see-through plastic, leather and velvet. Many online retailers have beginners' strap-on kits that are terrific.

Harnesses come in two general styles: a single-strap that is worn like a G-string panty and two-strap models, which have two straps running from the pubic bone, along the crease between the inner thigh and genitals, underneath the buttocks, and attach to the waistband in back. Some prefer the G-string style, saying it's a very stable base for the dildo and that it rubs the clit nicely when thrusting; others complain of getting a rash from the center string rubbing on their anus and tailbone. Another complaint about the G-string style is that it limits access to the wearer's genitals, so if a girl wanted to be penetrated or to massage her clit, it would be difficult. Also, they're not adaptable for male wearers.

Two-strap harnesses allow for plenty of genital access so wearers (of any gender) can masturbate or penetrate themselves, or be penetrated by another, while wearing the harness. For instance, a girl can fuck your G-spot while rubbing her clit or fucking herself with a dildo at the same time.

You'll also face choices when selecting a harness as to how the dildo is attached to or worn in the harness. Some strap-ons will have a simple hole in the middle, where the dildo is pulled through from the inside; while these are the easiest to get dildos in and out of, it's a "one size fits most" hole that will have smaller dildos sliding around and make bigger dildos difficult (or impossible) to squeeze in. Versatile harnesses have four straps that come through a triangular base and attach to a removable rubber O-ring in the center. This style provides the most stable base for a dildo and different O-ring sizes are available for purchase (many of these harnesses ship with three ring sizes), and cleanup is easy.

Make sure your harness fits right. The straps should be tight enough to withstand thrusting, but not so tight they pinch or cut into your skin; give the dildo a few tugs to see how it feels. The dildo shouldn't slip out, or around too much (though a little movement is fine). The dildo should rest right on or just above your pubic bone; if you get sore from thrusting you can buy a specially made pad of thin foam to cushion your pubic bone.

Sex Positions for G-Spot Stimulation

G-spot stimulation during penetration (penis or strap-on) requires a bit of coordination, but if you keep in mind where you're aiming, and put pressure in the right place during your strokes, it's just a matter of stamina! There are also a couple of sex positions that can make rubbing her spot a lot easier.

Foremost, remember that you'll be concentrating your efforts on the tip of whatever tool you're using; the cockhead is the primary massage tool here. Try using the tip to rub, massage and roll the G-spot area around. Read the massage techniques in the G-spot massage section for thrusting ideas to try out with your cock (be it flesh or silicone), and experiment with the following sex positions:

- *Woman on top:* this has her controlling the angle and pressure. She can lean back for more G-spot stimulation.
- *Doggy-style:* on all fours she can angle her hips (sometimes with the help of pillows) to get the right sensations while you thrust.
- *On her back:* she can put pillows under her hips to elevate her pussy, tilting it up or down with more pillows as it feels right for her.

Found

ALISON TYLER

O ne of the greatest pleasures about my job is the amount of time I get to spend on the road. I enjoy staying at different hotels, sometimes making up fantasy lives for myself, which I share, willingly, with people I meet at hotel bars. I adore living out of a suitcase because my business puts me up in the nicest accommodations. At home, I have a very small studio apartment with a loft for my bed and a tiny refrigerator. My bathroom is clean and decorated entirely in white. I have a shower stall but no bath-tub, something I'd never missed until this trip.

I'd spent the entire evening in the hotel bar, being chatted up by a very attractive man who struck me as slightly dangerous. Usually, I go for dangerous. If you saw me, you'd understand why. For my job, I am forced to wear conservative business suits, no-nonsense heels, and subdued jewelry. My short, red hair is always carefully coiffed. My perfume, when I wear any at all, is as understated as early morning fog.

Slightly dangerous men are absolutely my type, and absolutely the wrong kind of men to pick up when I am in a strange city on business. I knew that if I invited the handsome dark-eyed stranger back to my room I would get no work done at all and I'd have circles under my eyes when I met with two very important clients in the morning.

Instead, I demurred to his request that I let him show me the town, paid my tab, and, extremely aware of my damp panties, rode the elevator alone to my suite on the top floor. Once inside the room, I quickly rummaged through my suitcase, searching for my favorite toy. My fingers were trembling as they closed around the lavender, dolphin-shaped dildo. I needed to come, badly. I flicked on the switch with one hand, yanking my nylons and panties down with the other.

Nothing happened.

That's not to say that my cunt wasn't drippy wet, that my mind wasn't desperately regretting the fact that I'd left the rebel at the bar rather than allowing him up to my room. But nothing happened with my vibrator. The toy clicked, but the motor didn't hum to life. I checked the battery: nothing there. As luck would have it, I had forgotten the single most important accessory for a vibrator: fresh batteries. This may seem an inconsequential event to those less horny than I, but to me, the situation was traumatic. I called room service, only to be courteously told that I could purchase batteries in the gift shop when it opened in the morning at 8:30.

Christ, I couldn't wait seven hours.

I couldn't wait seven minutes.

I thought about using my fingers, but it's difficult and frustrating for me to get off that way. I'm in tune to the rhythm of my vibrator. For solo occasions, I don't really like much else.

Momentarily dumbstruck, I sat on the edge of the bed, contemplating calling down to the bar and trying to describe the dark horse who had so rudely stolen my peace of mind. But instead, flashing on an image from adolescence, I walked into the bathroom, shedding clothes on the way.

The hotel room boasted a large, sunken tub of pure white porcelain. I climbed in and slid my legs up to the rim, bending them at the knee and parting them as wide as they would go. Slowly, I turned on the faucet with one foot, maneuvering the temperature toward lukewarm. I felt those first few drops of water splash against my cunt, and I relaxed.

This was heaven.

I closed my eyes and leaned back in the tub. I hadn't put the stopper in, so I knew I wouldn't drown. The water dripped gently over me and then drained away. I pictured my bar mate, imagining I was experiencing his knowing tongue bringing me pleasure instead of the insistent homemade waterfall from the silver faucet. As I fantasized, I used my foot to nudge the temperature up slightly, building toward my climax by strengthening the water pressure and fooling with the hot and the cold.

My short hair was growing damp and the cold porcelain was taking on the heat of the water. I relaxed even more, using two fingers now on my pulsing clit, raising myself up as high as I could toward that glorious flow. I didn't need a dangerous man to keep me up at night. I didn't need the bite marks he would leave or the bruises on my pale skin. I only needed the faucet, the water, the tub, and my twisted and very active imagination.

As soon as I came, I turned off the water, wrapped myself in a towel, and headed toward the bed. I was actually mentally congratulating myself for avoiding temptation when I heard the knock.

What on earth? It was 2:00 a.m.

I tiptoed to the door and peered out into the hall, coming almost eye to eye with the stunner from the bar. How had he found my room number? How had he known that I'd just climaxed while envisioning him climbing between my thighs and licking my pussy? My cheeks turned as red as my hair. Yet all thoughts of being good disappeared. I unlocked the chain and opened the door, and in he came: a rush of energy, a force to behold. He kicked the door shut behind him, then backed me up against the bed, pulling my white terry cloth towel away from my still damp body, pressing himself insistently against me.

"You didn't really mean no, did you?"

"No..." I said, not sure what I had meant in the bar, or what I meant now. He took another step forward, pushing me onto the mattress.

"When you paid your tab, I saw your room number on the check. I've been pacing in my room, wondering whether to call or just come. I decided to come."

"I already did," I confessed, as his hand slid down my body to my cunt. I wondered if he could smell my arousal, if his fingers could sense the power of the orgasm I'd just had. He slid one finger between my slick nether lips and then all the way inside of me, laughing when he found the wetness awaiting him.

"And what did you think about when you came?"

I flushed darker still. "You."

"Me doing what?" He had me on my back now, and a second finger had joined his first. Slowly, he started to stroke me on the inside, and I suddenly found speaking difficult. Speaking English, anyway. Moaning was something I could do just fine. Wordless, begging moans escaped my lips as he began to touch me in a way nobody ever had.

What was he doing to me?

Those decadent fingers of his, fingers I'd admired when they were gripping the neck of his bottle of beer, were now hooked within me, massaging, probing.

But suddenly I pushed him away.

"I'm going to—"

"No," he said, "you just think you are. Relax into it. The feeling will pass. I promise."

I stared at him. How had he known? His eyes focused on mine. Maybe he didn't care if I did wet the bed. Maybe he was just that kind of a kinky part-ner. My breathing sped up as he continued to trick his fingers within me. He had found a spot, a place to work; compressing the flesh, kneading me; and he was right about one thing. In seconds, the need to pee had completely disappeared, while a whole different urgent yearning took over as the number-one craving within me.

The pillows were soft under my head and I arched my back, hips in the air, as he worked me relentlessly. I couldn't believe he'd found me, and I couldn't believe I was this turned on after just having come. Usually, I need a bit of downtime between orgasms to regain my sense of self.

But the handsome man at my side was giving me no chance to recover. God, he knew what he was doing. Firmly stroking, not tentative. Not hesitant at all.

"Tell me what you thought of," he murmured, "when you made yourself come."

I started to say "You," once more, but he shook his head. Clearly, he wanted details, not one-word answers.

"I pictured you bent down between my thighs," I told him softly, "licking my clit." A shiver rushed through me. "And then moving into a sixty-nine so that I could suck you, too."

As I spoke, he seemed to find the perfect rhythm, because suddenly I was on the verge. "Oh, Jesus," I hissed between my teeth. "Oh, god."

"Don't hold back," he demanded, but I couldn't have if I'd tried. His fingertips were magic within me, and in seconds I was coming again, more fiercely than before, the bed shaking with the motions of my hips on the mattress.

The handsome stranger didn't stop. He kept touching me through the whole violent ride of my orgasm, sucking in his breath at the abundance of the juices that wet his hand.

I thought I'd experienced a waterfall of pleasure in the tub. But this was different. A gush of liquid coated my pussy lips, my inner thighs, and my new partner's hand to the wrist. Nothing like this had ever happened to me before. Yes, I come hard, but I'd never come wet.

"What did you do to me?" I whispered as he started to take off his clothes.

"I found you," he said, eyes glowing.

"What do you mean?"

"You were looking for something tonight, weren't

you? Down there in the bar, flirting with me. You were looking. But I found you." He said the four words slowly, with meaning. And when I looked into his eyes, I thought I saw an echo of myself. Of the needs that make me who I am. Maybe traveling solo wasn't quite as exciting as it had been when I first started working. Maybe I was looking not only for a dangerous man to liven up my night—but one to invigorate my life.

He was naked then, and moving his body into the position I'd described to him, clicking his tongue against me gently as he lowered his hard cock to my lips.

And I let him. As I imagined letting him do so many other decadent things in the future.

chapter 5

wet spots: ejaculation

Female ejaculation has to be one of the most mis-understood sexual responses in history. Even though there's been significant research about what it is and where it comes from, the information is so rarely shared or disseminated that most people—even smart girls—don't know what it is. Or how it feels. Or if it's even okay to have happen to you.

Well, it's more than okay. Simply speaking, female ejaculation is when you have a powerful orgasm that pushes fluid from the many tiny glands and ducts that comprise the body of the G-spot. The fluid is clear and odorless, and it can be just a little bit or a lot. It's not pee. And many women say it feels really, really good to ejaculate.

In most cases, ejaculation happens as a result of G-spot stimulation. But a number of women can also ejaculate from clitoral orgasms, or vaginal penetration leading to orgasm—even when they weren't directly stimulating their G-spots. That's not to say that if you play with your G-spot, eventually you will have a gushing ejaculation; it's possible you might love, love, love coming with your G-spot, and yet never ejaculate. Women who don't easily ejaculate often have to consciously learn how to squirt—if they want to.

Not all women ejaculate, and not all care to. It's a matter of taste, your body's inclination to do so (though you can train yourself to squirt, not all women are successful at it), and whether or not you like the sensation. Not all women do. Some like it a lot, though, enough for it to become their preferred method of orgasm. These girls not only like it for the intensity that it can bring to their orgasms, but because they, and their lovers, love to see, feel, and experience these really wet and intense orgasms.

It's quite common to discover by accident that you can ejaculate—often, it happens when you come really hard and soak the bed (or your surprised lover). Because lots of girls have no idea what female ejaculation is, and that it's totally normal, their first natural reaction is surprise, embarrassment, or even shame. Shame, especially if you're worried it might be urine, or your lover doesn't know anything about female ejaculation and thinks you wet yourself. Well, you didn't. And don't ever let anyone tell you that you did. Also, don't be fooled by the myth that once you start to squirt, you won't be able to stop—this simply isn't true, as you'll understand after reading the following sections on muscle control and the physiological ejaculatory process.

Granted, not all women have this reaction; oodles of girls try in earnest to learn how to ejaculate successfully, and often their partners try really hard to help them squirt when they come. Also, a good number of girls discover as they hone their individual orgasm style that ejaculation is just part of their wet and wonderful orgasmic process; it's what they've always done, and they have no problems with it, thank you very much.

Think of female ejaculation as being your own awesome orgasmic superpower. To the untrained eye, you're a regular girl. But to those you trust, and those who deserve it, your pussy is like Wonder Woman. When you've had enough fun getting turned on and coming in the ways of mortal girls, you can unleash an orgasm your lovers can see, feel, taste and never, ever forget.

What's Going On Here?

When you have a G-spot orgasm accompanied by ejaculation, not only has your G-spot come alive, but

so also have all the tissues, glands and ducts surrounding the entire area. The spongy tissues that
surround your urethra and comprise your G-spot
make up quite a system. You have the erectile tissue
I described at length in chapter 2, and you've also
got the nerve-rich urethra itself and about forty
super-tiny glands and ducts (called, you'll remember, paraurethral glands, or Skene's glands) that
respond to arousal and pleasure. When you come hard
and ejaculate, there is an expulsion of fluid from the
urethral sponge and ducts, and the paraurethral
glands are what's responsible.

When you see an ejaculation—in person, or in
authentic "squirting" porn—you'll see the entire area
around the urethra swell up, big-time. When the
moment of orgasm happens, you'll see the whole area
get super-puffy and darken in color. At the apex,
you'll be able to see the muscles contract and the
whole area distinctly looking like it's bearing down
to push out squirt after squirt of watery liquid.
Sometimes the force and range of the fluid coming
out is pretty surprising—there's obviously a lot of
power behind what's going on here.

The ejaculate itself is what's called prostatic-like
fluid, meaning that the glands pushing fluid out of
the little ducts are prostate-like; the fluid contains
some elements similar to what's found in prostatic

fluids in men. Again, the fluid is not urine, though some evaluations have shown small, trace amounts of urine in female ejaculate, presumably because the exit point is also where urine leaves the body. The fluid does not come from, or pass through the bladder. It's clear and watery, scentless, slightly slippery (though useless as lubrication, as the slipperiness doesn't last), and some people say it has a slightly sweet taste.

Amazingly, women who ejaculate are often able to do it more than once. And in copious amounts. The amount of fluid expelled upon orgasm can be anywhere from a teaspoon to one and a half cups (!) of ejaculate, and mega-squirting girls can do these big loads multiple times, sometimes two or three in a row, one after another. Needless to say, this is the type of activity for which staying hydrated is essential.

How to Ejaculate

If you want to ejaculate, all you need to do is get in shape and practice. Sounds fun, doesn't it? Women who ejaculate freely, on demand, and with style, typically have really excellent PC (pubococcygeus) muscles. This means that the whole sling of muscles that line your pelvis, and especially those that play

How to Stop

It's one thing to want to ejaculate and to teach your body how, but some girls want just the opposite—they want a break from all the gushing orgasms, or just to be able to turn it off and on easier. The answer in both of these situations lies in PC muscle tone: the stronger and more toned your PCs are, the more control you'll have. So get those muscles in shape.

starring roles in your orgasmic process, are in great shape. They're toned, responsive, and strong. And for most of us, this doesn't just happen. Having good PC muscle tone means getting them in shape, which means exercising them. And there are a lot of really fun ways to do this—and no one need be the wiser when you "work out."

If you're not sure where your PC muscles are, let alone how to pump them up, there are two easy ways to isolate them. One is to stop a stream of pee mid-flow; next time you're urinating, halt the pee for a second. Those are the muscles you'll want to learn how to flex. Another way to find the same muscles is to insert a finger (or fingers), or a firm sex toy, into your vagina and squeeze hard. The object will provide enough resistance for you to feel those muscles push, and if you're using a finger you'll be able to feel your muscles close down around your finger.

Getting your PC muscles in shape is a snap, and unlike other workout routines, you can customize your PC exercises to fit your lifestyle. For instance, you can set aside time once a day, or every other day, to practice with a toy. Many women swear by a toy that is basically a heavy "vaginal barbell," made of steel and sold at sex toy boutiques. The Kegelcisor and Betty's Barbell are the most recognized name brands, but you can use other toys that work just the same (and cost less), made of glass or plastic. The firmness and weight of toys like the barbell provide excellent resistance for squeezing and making your muscles strong; many women find doing these exercises particularly arousing, just because of the way they "wake up" the entire genital area.

Truly, any hard toy will do for your PC reps; another gadget some women really like is the Kegelmaster, a device that actually reads and registers your PC muscle strength, letting you know how you're progressing. Ignore the "as seen on TV" marketing hype and you've got an interesting tool for providing resistance to increase vaginal tone and orgasmic strength.

Even though some women prefer to use a toy for PC exercises, many women get great results from

rhythmically squeezing their PC muscles *without* a
toy—mostly because we can do this anywhere, any-
time, whenever we remember, and no one can even
tell what we're doing. With or without a toy, your
goal is to squeeze your PC muscles in a variety of different ways, repetitively and regularly. Try once a day,
twice a day, or several sets every other day. Toning
your PC muscles does more than help you become a
squirter; it'll help you control the squirting, make
your orgasms stronger, increase your pelvic health,
and increase healthy blood flow to your entire genital system.

Here are a few workout suggestions for reps you
can repeat in sets or cycle through as you like:

- Squeeze, hold, release. Repeat ten times.
- Squeeze in rapid pulses, ten to fifteen times in
  a row.
- Tense your PC muscles; hold for a deep inhale
  and exhale.
- Repeat the above techniques, but with a distinct
  sense of bearing down, or pushing outward.
- Repeat the same exercises, pulling inward, as
  if holding something in or trying to pull something inside you.
- See how many repetitions you can do in a row.
  100? 200?

Ejaculation Techniques

Learning to squirt requires formulating your own individual means of getting there, much like finding the ways you like to come when you masturbate. Overall, though, most women who ejaculate can agree that when they are at the point of gushing, bearing down or pushing is what gets them to their slippery destination. For some it's a conscious effort to actually push the ejaculate out; others say that they just feel like they have to press outward, almost involuntarily, as if they were coming outwardly, rather than the kind of orgasmic pulsing that feels like inward contractions.

Often, you might find that bearing down or needing to push with your pussy makes it difficult to squirt with anything in there, like a penis, fingers, a fist or a toy. You'll get yourself up to the point of having to come, then feel the need to push, and whatever was in your vagina to get you to the apex had better get the hell out of the way! Conversely, there may also be times when you'll want to keep whatever got you to the brink of orgasm right where it is, to take you over the edge, using the toy or person as the focus of your orgasmic efforts.

Here are some tips for successful ejaculation:

- Pee first.

- Some women find that it's easier to squirt if they've already had an orgasm—or two.
- Use a vibrator on your clit, or a vibrating G-spot toy if it turns you on more.
- Stimulate your G-spot until you feel like you're going to come.
- You might feel like you have to pee for a second, and then it subsides. You don't have to pee, but you're getting close to squirting.
- Relax.
- Keep playing with your G-spot, and tilt your hips up, like a pelvic thrust. When you thrust, push with your PC muscles for a second. Then go back to G-spot massage in a resting position—then repeat.
- When you're about to come, thrust and push while jacking your G-spot as hard as you like it. Don't worry—you can't hurt yourself jacking off like this, no matter how big the object (or fist) is, or how hard you're pressing.
- Try different positions: on your back, seated in a chair, standing, or doggy-style.
- Don't fret if you don't come. Maybe you will next time, maybe you will a few more times from now, maybe you'll decide not to squirt at all. It's all fun; just experiment with feeling good and seeing what your body likes.

- If you do ejaculate, see if you can do it again!
- When you're done, go pee again to clear out your bladder, just as you would after any other sexual activities.

Wet Spots and Creative Solutions

This is a wet sport. No doubt about it; if you ejaculate, you're going to make a mess. But what a delightful, delicious and delirious mess it is. Your sheets will get soaked, sometimes your mattress too—and if you're out of bed, you'll leave your slippery orgasmic evidence wherever you came. That's not a bad thing at all, it just means that squirting orgasms will require a bit of forethought, much more than a finger-in-the-panties, clitoral quickie.

Like I said earlier, you might emit a bit of fluid—or a lot. If it's minimal, you'll just want to have a towel handy for afterward, and expect to maybe leave a little spot every now and then. But if you're one of the many women who ejaculate copious amounts of come, then you'll want to have towels (plural) at the ready, beneath your hips or your lover's, or out in front of whatever direction you have your G-spot aimed.

If you're a bed-soaker, invest in some lined sheets (like ones used in cribs); or thick, inexpensive mattress pads that you won't mind washing every time you come. You can also pick up a product called Luv Liners, absorbent, disposable waterproof pads that are made especially for adults who enjoy messy sex moments. Of course, you can always try to get it all over your lover, making for a seriously sexy "come in his face" (or on her chest) moment—or you can be even more premeditated and have sex in the bathtub, on tiled surfaces that clean up easily (like those in the kitchen), or outdoors.

Down to Business

ALISON TYLER

W e should stop," you say in that semisweet, semismug tone of yours. "Really, we should." I can tell from the taunting look in your lovely large eyes exactly how you want me to respond. I don't need any additional hints, but you continue as if I do. "It's against the rules," you add, gazing down at the floor as if shocked by your own naughty behavior.

"What is?" I ask, softly. "This?"

"Oh, yes," you tell me, playing coy now. "That's just wrong, wrong, wrong."

Now, I press you up against the wall of your office so that your palms are splayed flat on the wood-paneled wall. Then I slide that short black skirt up past your curvaceous hips. I take my time, because I like to admire the view. "Or this?" I whisper, my mouth against your neck, teeth poised and ready to bite. You can feel my hot breath on your skin and that makes you tremble.

"That," you insist. "That's just flat-out unacceptable."

"Ah," I sigh. "This is all getting clearer to me. You're saying that I'm just not supposed to do this—" As I speak, I gently slip your lilac satin panties aside. I love these panties. The black lace trim is a total turn-on, and the way they perfectly and snugly fit your ass drives me wild. I know that you wore them for me, and that thought makes me even harder. You looking through all of the naughty knickers in your collection before choosing this particular set is an image I adore.

Even though I do love occasionally absconding with your panties, slipping them into a jacket pocket to take home and play with later—this afternoon, I don't take them down; just push the smooth, slippery fabric out of my way, and my fingertips play out an immediate melody over your clit. For a moment, I make you lose your cool. My fingers stroke and tap, and you suck in your breath at the first wave of pleasure.

You can't be so clever now, can you? Not as the shining wetness coats my fingers, as I raise back up and stand next to you, staring directly at you as I lick your juices off the tips.

"Oh, god," you groan. You can't suppress the shudder that throbs through you as you watch. Don't you love the way that looks? Me slowly, so slowly, tonguing away your sweet nectar?

"Is this wrong?" I ask, reaching my hand up under your skirt again to collect a fresh dose of your honeyed juices on the tips of my fingers. The first taste of you has made me hungry for more.

"No, don't stop—"

At your request, my fingers probe deeper, and I hold on to you with one hand, keeping you steady as I finger-fuck that sweet pussy of yours. I want you to be ripe and ready for me by the time I take my cock out. You need all the lubrication you can get, because I'm going to fuck you good. Even harder than you're thinking about right now. I'm going to slam you up against the wall and make you forget how to be coy. How to tease me with those bedroom eyes of yours. Or should I call them 'boardroom eyes'?

"I don't know," I say, dropping onto my knees and bringing my face right up to your cunt. I breathe in, adoring the smell of your sex. The scent makes me dizzy with need. "If employees aren't supposed to date, then you probably shouldn't let me lick your pussy."

"Doesn't say anything about that—" you assure me in a rush.

"What do you mean?" I tease. "What are you implying? That we should sidestep the rules? That wouldn't be fair to the rest of the workforce, would it?"

"I'm just saying—" you start, but then you can't finish your thought because my tongue is already tripping along the seam of your body, playing you so sweetly. I know how to take care of you. I know the little tricks that you like best. My tongue makes several smooth rotations right around your clit, not actually touching that hot little gem, just brushing around it carefully. Slowly. And then, right when you think you're going to die if I don't touch you where you want, I slide my tongue along your clit in one long brushstroke. You grip my hair and hold on, shivering, so close already that I'm sure you can imagine exactly how good it's going to feel when I let you come. But I'm not letting you. Not yet. With a slow and steady pace, I resume those lazy, crazy, everlasting circles that make you want to sprawl out on the plushly carpeted floor and let me just lick you for hours.

"So," I say, speaking right up against your most tender skin. "What would page ten have to say about this—?"

"No, nothing, nothing," you whisper, and it sounds as if you're begging. You're the one who brought it up, though. Remember that when I make you bite down on your lip to stifle your screams of pleasure. *You're* the one who opened the manual and used a bright lemon-yellow highlighter pen to illuminate all the different rules that we were breaking.

"What about this?" I tease, standing up next to you once more, driving my fingers inside of you as I search within. You groan when I curl my fingertips forward, finding that spot that makes you weak. I have to flip you around once more, holding you up against the wall with one hand as I press deep into your pussy, working you just right.

If I touch you the way you need, I'll make you gush. I've never been with a woman before who climaxed the way you do. You don't just get wet, you come like a fountain. I see you squeeze your eyelids shut tight as the pressure starts to build. You make a soft keening noise deep in your throat, and I can tell you're lost. There will be no more talk about rules. There will be only pleasure.

The first time we played like this, you swore you were going to wet yourself. But I just kept going, not stopping for a second. Make a puddle on my floor? Who the fuck cares? You didn't. You started to moan and purr. And then you started to come, shocking me with the intensity of your orgasm while my fingers continued to press against that special spot inside of you. You wet your thighs and my face and the sheets beneath us. And afterward, you were embarrassed, as if something had gone wrong.

But everything had gone right. So fucking right.

Now, it's my goal every time. Now, I revel in the encounters we have in which I can get you to this point. Where you shiver all over. Where you actually manage to ejaculate. Where you have to go in search of your spare panties and hose tucked away in your filing cabinet to replace the ones dampened by our lust.

I can tell now that you're dangerously close, and I keep up my efforts, touching harder now, touching you the way you need. The palm of my hand cradles your clit as my fingers rotate over your G-spot, pressing, teasing. I've gotten good over the last few months. I can find that area without so much trouble, my fingertips homing in on it.

Suddenly, you start to tremble.

Coming like this makes you weak-kneed. The climax doesn't subside like a normal clitoral orgasm. This type rolls through you in waves, shaking you from the inside out with the pleasure of a thousand small orgasms linked together. You've tried to explain the way you feel, and I've listened in awe, wishing I could climb inside of you, experience the firework explosions that you whisper to me about afterward.

I revel in the vision, watching you lose control, and then, when I can't wait another damn second, I remove my hand and flip you around despite your whimper of protest, and I push against you.

This is my favorite way to fuck, driving in from behind with both of us standing, but at first I simply let you feel my cock against you through my clothes. I want you to know precisely how excited I am. How ready I am for you. When you whimper again, I rip open my fly and pull out my rod. You're in the perfect position, back arched, poised to receive me. I wrap one hand around your mane of dark hair and tilt your head back so that I can watch your face as I slide inside you. That first deep push is unlike any other sensation. The way your body surrounds me is sublime.

Your body is still trying to absorb the pleasure of your initial climax. Your cunt grips me, milks me, and I'm lost almost from the very start.

You've got yourself under control now, but I can see the sheen on your skin. Your body is hungry for more.

God, are you lovely. Your eyes, which grew wider at the moment of penetration, now get a faraway look, as if you've just arrived at some wonderful distant location. That exotic location called "I've almost reached it." We both know all about that place. And I'm going to take you even further—to a tropical island called "coming together."

Out in the hall I can hear the bustle of secretaries working. Hear the voices and the sounds of their fingers on the keyboards. Their chitchat on the telephones. I hear the low, gruff talk as different employees hurry past the room. Everyone's busy. Everyone needs something. Nobody will bother us, though. That's not even a tiny worry on my radar screen. Officially, we're holding a meeting, the two of us—an important, private meeting—so we can take our time.

Our time to do all the things I need to do to you. And I need to do so many things. Rutting forward. Driving hard. I need to make you crazy with the fact that you can't make noise. You can't be loud.

I want you to be warm and pliant, relaxed and ready, for what we're going to do next. Because this is what I think about it all, baby—if we're going to break those boundaries, we might as well do it right. Might as well really get down to business.

Don't you agree?

faster, deeper, more!

Now that you've discovered G-spot play and those crazier, stronger orgasms, what are you going to do with your supercharged pussy? Just as if you'd been handed the keys to a brand-new hot rod, you're probably going to want to see what this thing can do, and how many ways you can combine it with all kinds of other sex play, like anal sex, oral sex and more. You might even find that you like more intense penetration, or fullness (like from a fist), or a variety of sensations—like pain or heat or sensory deprivation—during G-spot play.

G-Spot Play with Vibrators

For many women, their preferred style of G-spot play will include toys, and as we saw in chapter

3, there's lots of variety to choose from. Many toys involve some sort of use of vibration to stimulate. Vibration is conducive to many a G-spot orgasm: you may like the feeling of a vibrator only on your clit, on the G-spot itself, or just in the whole general area of your vaginal entrance. Strong buzz or soft, a vibrator will feel intense (intensely good) around your clit, your outer and inner labia, and inside the vaginal opening. But as far as sensation goes, the vibration won't matter so much once it's inside; the size, shape, and movement of the vibrator will.

Here are a few tips to consider if you're operating a sex toy for someone else's G-spot pleasure:

- Always start with a vibrator's lowest speed, and give her more as she asks for it.
- Remember to never put a vibe directly on sensitive areas like the clit or G-spot right away; always start from the side.
- With any toy, vibrating or not, give her just what she wants—and then a little bit more. Caress and knead her labia and clit, and build up to penetration (unless she demands otherwise).
- Once inside, focus the tip of the toy around her G-spot area, massaging it on the in stroke, or out stroke, or both.

- You can hold the toy stationary, allowing her to control the stimulation with her hip movements.

G-Spot Play with Anal Sex

G-spots and butt plugs go together like lips and kisses. In fact, anal penetration is a wonderful sensory complement to G-spot massage, creating a wide range of deliciously strong sensations all in one area. If you like anal sex, and you love your G-spot, then you'll want to invest in some high-quality butt toys, or enlist a lucky lover to play with your ass while you play with your G-spot—or vice versa, or you can just let him or her run rampant with your happy orifices. As a primer for anal play, always follow these rules: go very slowly, listen to the person you're penetrating (or check in with yourself), and use lots of lube. Only start anal stimulation when you're aroused; otherwise, it might not feel so good. Anal penetration hurts when you go too fast, you don't use enough lube, you're not relaxed, or you really aren't in the mood.

Anal play isn't for everyone, so if you want to play with your girl's butt in combination with G-spot play, be sure to cover the topic with her before you go anywhere near her ass. See if she wants to start playing with her butt before, during or after G-spot stimulation so you know when to begin.

Butt Basics

Much like the vagina, the outer third of the anus (and, in men, the prostate) contains more nerve endings than the anal canal and responds best to touch and vibration. The inner portion, inside the canal, has fewer nerve endings near the skin's surface and responds more to feelings of fullness, pressure, and rhythm.

The anus has really thin skin, and while it may not be sensitive to insults, it can damage easily from even the tiniest scratchy surface or hangnail, and even rough skin on the hands can make it feel uncomfortable or irritated. Be absolutely sure that anything you massage or insert into the rectum is totally smooth, especially plastic sex toys. Lubricant can ease most surface tension and discomfort from friction, and because the anus does not self-lubricate (like a vagina), you'll need to be heavy-handed with that bottle of lube.

Squirt liberal amounts of lube onto any toy you use, and reapply frequently. Sex toys used for anal penetration must have a flared base, meaning a base that prevents them from being pulled into the anal canal, where they can get lost—a nightmare waiting to happen. The sphincter muscles squeeze and contract as they please; we cannot completely control them. This serves to push and pull things in and out of the anus, and once something gets pulled in, there's no guarantee you're going to get it out without a trip to the hospital—which is what you'd have to do to prevent serous injury if, say, a hot, battery-powered vibrator went AWOL. Take a look at a standard butt plug and you'll see exactly what a flared base should look like.

Much like G-spot play, anal enjoyment is best begun when you're already turned on—and some women prefer to have an orgasm before even thinking about having any backdoor adventures. Getting turned on beforehand is key to relaxing the muscles and making you receptive to trying more intense sensations, and continuing pleasurable stimulation (like clitoral or G-spot play) during anal penetration is a tried-and-true technique many women use to get off during anal sex. Start aroused, go very slow, use lots of lube and stay relaxed. Anal penetration might feel a bit uncomfortable for a minute, but it should never hurt. Again, if it hurts, then you're going too fast, you need more lube, you're not turned on enough, or you're really not in the mood.

Getting Started with Anal Penetration

If you're new to anal penetration, start with the flat pad of your finger or the side of your sex toy's tip, press lightly on the opening, and hold it there. A lot of people find that vibrators make butt play easier, especially for beginners, so you might want to get a butt toy that vibrates. Anal vibration feels incredible during G-spot play. Be sure to stimulate yourself (clit or G-spot) the entire time you're playing with your ass. Increase the pressure on your anus a little at a time, massaging and pressing in circular motions. Go slow—for some girls, simply having it touched during G-spot stimulation feels plenty good, and could be enough for an orgasm. Use lots of lube, even if you don't go in yet: don't rely on saliva at all.

Move your toy in a circular motion, and begin experimenting with penetration by pressing in a little bit more. If you're using fingers, make sure that you've clipped your fingernails down and filed them totally smooth, or use a latex glove or finger cot to make your finger a perfectly smooth surface. When you're ready, slide your toy or finger in up to the first joint (about an inch), and hold it there for a few breaths. Keep up the G-spot (or clitoral) stimulation as you penetrate yourself. You'll feel the ring of muscles around your anal opening squeeze and contract; just stay still as they relax.

When you feel your muscles relax, slide your toy or finger in a little bit more, and back out, doing a gentle in and out. If it feels good and you want more, you can go deeper and faster, add more fingers, turn on vibration, have your lover take over, or use a bigger toy. Also, once you're warmed up your lover can have anal sex with you while you use a toy on your G-spot: missionary, doggy-style, and woman-on-top are great positions for this style of double penetration.

Try inserting a butt plug and keeping it in place while you bring yourself to a G-spot orgasm. Butt plugs are also terrific to put in place during partnered G-spot sex—they keep the anal pleasure up while your lover thrusts against your G-spot. Chances are good that your PC muscles will squeeze the plug out before or during orgasm; you can ask your lover to hold it in place with his or her hand. But if it's big and stays in place, after you come, take a few deep breaths and then remove it on the second or third exhale.

G-Spot Play with Oral Sex

Cunnilingus is particularly well-suited for mixing it up with G-spot play; it's superfun to lick, suck and bring her off clitorally with your mouth as you stimulate her G-spot with your fingers or a toy. The easiest way will be to tilt your head to one side while you lick, moving your chin out of the way for better access to her vaginal opening.

Keep the basics of cunnilingus in mind when you're going down on her and playing with her spot simultaneously. The clit is very sensitive, like the G-spot; don't dive for it, but instead massage the sides until she's aroused enough for direct stimulation. Watch her physical cues—if she seems to be inching away from you, you're probably in the right spot, but putting too much pressure or moving too fast: ask her what she wants as often as possible. (You can read about cunnilingus techniques in detail in my book *The Ultimate Guide to Cunnilingus*.)

When she gets really turned on and nears orgasm, you'll be putting a lot of pressure on her clit with your tongue, and massaging her G-spot quite firmly. She'll likely be bucking into your face pretty hard— be prepared for hand and neck pressure or strain! When she's about to come, don't stop or switch any of your techniques—just ride the same pressure, rhythm and motion through until she's done.

If she's an ejaculator, you'll want to make a decision beforehand as to whether or not you want her to come in your face or mouth. Think about what would be okay for you, and if you don't mind (or it turns you on), great. But if you'd rather not get a face full of her come, you can angle your head sideways and up to avoid the stream, or lean back completely as she comes; you can have it spray on your chest or arm; you could even lay your head on her pubic area and watch it spray out, with a view from her clit.

Spice up cunnilingus and G-spot play with the following sensory tricks:

- Get a bowl or cup of ice and put a cube in your mouth to cool down your tongue and lips.
- Use an iced or hot drink to change the temperature of your mouth. You'll know if it's too hot or cool because it will be uncomfortable for you, too. Pause while licking and take a mouthful of the beverage; swish and swirl it around your mouth for a minute, then swallow. Continue licking until you feel the temperature change, then repeat as necessary.
- Menthol and mint cough drops and breath mints are amazing cunnilingus sex toys. Look for lozenges with both menthol and mint (they're the strongest), and be sure to get sugar-free versions to avoid irritating her vaginal ecosystem. Before you go down, put one in your mouth and swish it around to activate it and soften the corners—you don't want a corner to accidentally scrape her clit. When you're good and mentholated, slip the lozenge between your cheek and gums. Putting it

under your tongue will make it pop out, and trying to rest it on the back of your tongue while you lick could make you choke on it, so don't do either of those. Add to the icy sensations by blowing softly on her vulva—and please, no puffing any air inside the vagina, as it can be potentially harmful.

G-Spot Play with S/M and Power Play

Do you like hot sauce? Some people do—some like it a lot—and liking the taste of good food accompanied by intense sensation is a great analogy for people who like pain with their pleasure. Sometimes a little spice will do, thank you, while at other times all you want is that mouth-on-fire, nose-running sensation from the wasabi at your favorite sushi bar or the salsa at the local burrito joint. For women who like a range of sensations (from mild to hot!), G-spot play is an ideal sexual activity for adding a little or a lot of pleasurable pain. Or the pain might be a side dish, acting as reward or punishment to your G-spot play power exchange session.

Always talk about pain, pleasure, dominance, submission and any kind of power exchange or sensation play before you do it—even if you think you "know" she'll be into it. Just make everything really clear; what she wants and likes, and how far you can go with any of your fun and games.

You can select from any number of ways to up the ante with G-spot play and intense sensations. The two of you may have decided that you want to add pain into your regular G-spot routine as if it were a sex toy, and simply experiment with techniques and toys. Or it could be that you have a fantasy scenario in mind in which one of you is dominant and the other submissive, and some spanking or rough play fuels the fantasy's fire. Perhaps you just want to play the dominant partner, and take rough control of her nipples and clit, or treat her stomach or breasts to clips and clamps or a light whipping as you stimulate her G-spot. She may simply enjoy the way pain adds to her G-spot sensations; or perhaps one particular thing pushes her over the edge, such as nipple biting upon orgasm, and role-play or fantasy don't enter into it at all. Pain, as a sex toy, can be shaped to fit your own personal sexual expression, just as G-spot stimulation will evolve naturally in its own pleasurable ways.

Play with her G-spot and add a variety of eye-opening sensations to the mix. A simple pussy-slapping on her clit and mons with one hand in between thrusts with the other can turn into an all-out spanking if you (and she) like—add a twist with her legs fastened securely apart. Get more intense by adding a leather or rubber slapper—available at S/M boutiques or higher-end sex toy stores. Massage her G-spot until she's blissed out, then begin a rapid or slow series of thwacks, then go back to pleasure. You can also use a small or medium-sized flogger to the same effect.

For adding pain to G-spot play, clips and clamps will be your best friends. Buy ones in specialty S/M boutiques or sex toy stores for this purpose; don't get ones with serrated tips. Place them on fleshy areas like nipples, breasts, arms, thighs, outer labia or stomach and then get to work on her G-spot. You can do much more with clips than just putting them on and taking them off: when the clips are on and you're working her spot, you can give her intense bursts of pain (and remind her the clips are still there) by merely touching the clips, pulling on the skin surrounding them, or even flicking them with your fingers. Pulling and twisting them hurts a lot, too. You don't have to confine your application to the outer labia; the inner labia and clitoris are open game if she's up for it, and licking around and on the clips can elicit a desirable response. Wrap rubber bands around larger clips such as clothespins to make them tighter, or to pull several together.

If your gal asks you to tie her up, and you have talked about what she'd like you to do, stimulating her G-spot when she's in such a helpless state may give her the most powerful orgasms she's ever had. A blindfold adds to the erotic intensity of feeling that she's under your control. With her sense of sight eliminated, she's forced to rely on her other senses, heightening all incoming stimuli, and she has to rely on you for direction. Plus, she can't see what you're up to, which simultaneously makes you more comfortable and her less steady.

You can blindfold her at any point, though some would argue that the sooner the games begin, the better. Try blindfolding her at the very beginning, and then proceed with your lovemaking as usual, even stripping her clothes off for her and making it all last as long as you can before you start massaging her G-spot. Or tell her that at some point, a point that you will determine, you will blindfold her and she will be under your control. If you've agreed on it, tie her up blindfolded and begin your G-spot ministrations on her fully bound and blind. It's a lot of fun to watch her respond unself-consciously.

G-Spot Play with a Fist

A significant number of women prefer their G-spot stimulation from fisting, and lots of women who ejaculate achieve their best come shots from fisting sessions. When someone is fisted, whether vaginally or anally, he or she receives penetration from her partner's entire hand, which is curled into a flexible, compact fist. For people who've never even contemplated penetration with larger objects, this sounds like it might hurt, and the term *fisting* makes it sound almost violent, as if there was punching involved. There isn't. And fisting, when done correctly with someone who likes it, doesn't hurt. In fact, for people who love the feeling of being "filled up," it can induce mind-blowing orgasms.

It's a very slow process that involves a lot of patience, a highly sexually aroused recipient, and a lot of lube. The person being fisted directs the action, instructing the penetrator as she goes along, telling her to add a finger, add rhythm, add lube, slow down, stop, or continue. The effect is a feeling of fullness or stretching, and since both the vaginal canal and the anal canal are elastic, they do not get "stretched out," and return to their previous size soon after orgasm.

Before even thinking of inserting your hand into your lover, take a close look and make sure your hands are perfectly clean and you have no jagged edges or cuts; if you're not sure, don a latex or nitrile (non-latex) glove. Gloves tend to feel smoother anyway, and she may prefer the sensation to the "drag" of your skin, especially if you have rough hands.

Before taking more than a few fingers, she'll need to be good and turned on—highly aroused and really excited about cramming as much of your hand into her as possible. Apply generous amounts of lube—water-based, thick gel is recommended—to your hand and her pussy. Go slowly into your normal fingering routine, as you insert one, two, three fingers inside. Her vaginal walls will be forming your fingers into the shape they want—sort of like a beak, with your fingers coming together at the tips. Let the shape of her pussy guide the shape of your hand—don't try to force your fingers straight or at any angle, but instead follow the natural curve of her vagina. Add more lube; keep everything very wet and messy.

Once you get your last finger in, slide your thumb underneath the fingers, completing the "beak" shape. Keep her engine revving; she could even be using a vibrator on her clit the entire time if she likes. Massage her pussy with your beaked hand; you'll feel her pussy push your hand into a loose fist shape once your knuckles start to slide past the opening. Your fingers will naturally want to curl over so the second finger joint is the tip of what's penetrating her.

Now what happens is really up to her. She might have had enough intense sensation; she may want you to very gently, slowly start to rock your fist a bit, or more. For many women, this will feel very intense, and you may notice that your slightest movements will be earthshaking for her. Other women will want more—and you'd better give it to them! Let her tell you—and show you—what she wants. She may want you to all-out fuck her with your fist; she might want to fuck herself at her own pace on your hand, like it's some kind of big, wet and wonderful sex toy.

Women who ejaculate will most likely want you to pump them up to the brink, and then pull out so they can squirt. Loosen and uncurl your fingers back into the loose beak shape as you slowly pull out; if she came and you're getting your hand back, you might ask her to take a few slow deep breaths, pulling it out on her last exhale. It might take a miniscule wiggle to get your knuckles past the muscles at the opening of her vagina—very similar to pulling a big butt plug past the ring of sphincter muscles that surround the anal opening. Then, of course, ask if she wants to do it again!

Pervert

ALISON TYLER

"Pretty girl," Charles says. "Who's my pretty girl?" I turn my head toward the wall and mumble an almost inaudible response.

"Can't hear you, love," he chides me. "Can't hear my girl."

"*I am*," I repeat, knowing that he's not looking at my face. Knowing that what he's referring to, what *he* thinks is pretty, is my pussy. That's where he is, right now, down there between my long legs, flash-light in one hand, industrial-size magnifying glass in the other.

He likes to look inside of me. He likes to turn off the lights in the bedroom, get in between my thighs, and shine a flashlight directly on my private parts. He says he's observing the intricacies of my cunt, the gradations of color—from pale petal to candy pink to darkest rose—the soft and subtle folds of skin. He watches and plays and remarks on the precise moment when I start to get dewy wet, when my hips begin to lift off the crisp navy-blue sheet and beg him, silently, wordlessly, to drop the flashlight and give me what I need.

Sometimes, we play doctor. He slides on a pair of thin ecru-colored rubber gloves. He gets the lube and the thermometer and sets everything up nice and neat on the bedside table. On these nights, he has me put on my old white nightgown backward, with the buttons running down my spine instead of the front. He pokes and prods, takes my temperature rectally, gives me a complete examination.

Other times, he simply observes, creating his own experiments, on the mission to make me come. To give me the best climax yet.

With a hand mirror, he shows me what I look like. He holds it between my legs and rotates the rounded glass so that I can see what he sees. Although I can't really see what he sees, not through his eyes. He points to my clit, gently lifting the hood of skin that covers it, making me tingle all over from the sensation of being brushed directly. I shift my hips on the mattress in an agony of yearning. It's more than I can take, that kind of stimulation, and I close my eyes and lie back against the pillows and beg, this time not so wordlessly, for him to give me what I want.

"Come on, Charlie. Please."

But no. Charlie takes things at his own speed. Never rush a doctor, he likes to say.

With the flashlight handy, he has me roll over, and he parts the cheeks of my ass. He rubs lubricant on my hole and probes me there with one finger, with two, watching the entire time under the glare from the mini-spotlight. It turns him on to feel my ass muscles squeeze on his fingers, but he admonishes me nonetheless, saying, "This is an examination, girl, don't get so excited."

But I *do* get excited, feeling slightly violated but worshipped just the same. All that attention, at close range, makes me desperately wet, which, in his clinical manner, he comments on, or records in a notebook he keeps specifically for this purpose.

Date: January 14th.
Time 9:45.
Notes: Patient responds with abundance of sexual juices when probed anally.

Sometimes, I'm screaming for him to fuck me by the end of the examination. Sometimes, I can't handle all the poking and prodding, and I just say, "Please, please, put it in me.... Charlie, come on, Charlie. Fuck me." But he takes his sweet time, getting close up to my ass and slipping three fingers inside, then four.

Once, when I couldn't wait another second, he fucked me with the cool, condom-clad metal handle of the flashlight, sliding it into my cunt, letting me grip on to the textured handle with the muscles of my pussy. With me so well-filled there, he decided that he needed to examine my asshole with something big: his cock. He was hard as the metal flashlight by this point, as excited by all his observations as I was. He filled me in back with his cock, and continued to fuck me with the tool. The light went off, and we were in the dark but didn't care, rocking on each other, jamming on each other.

But tonight is different.

Tonight he is on a discovery mission with a purpose.

Tonight, he wants to find my G-spot.

"I don't believe in it," I tell him. I've looked before. On a lonely night, all by myself, I tried with my own fingers to find that elusive little magic location. I'd read about G-spots in a magazine at the doctor's office. And I'd wanted to experience that otherworldly type of orgasm myself, the one described by the different interviewees. One woman had described experiencing near endless orgasms for an hour, her body rolling from one to the next. Another had said that clitoral climaxes were fine—but they were nothing astounding, nothing magnificent like a G-spot explosion.

Uselessly, I'd searched for that grape-sized area between the pubic bone and the cervix. I'd curled my fingers as the magazine described. And I didn't give up right away, either. *I'm a modern woman*, I told myself. *I should be responsible for my own pleasure.*

But I couldn't grasp what the fuss was about. I wanted to find it. I really did. And yet after what I felt was a full-on search, I ended up settling for a regular, run-of-the-mill climax. Not covering any new ground at all. Sure, no orgasm is bad, but I felt left out.

I should have known that Charles wouldn't let me off so easily. He has a manual. He has a flashlight. He's set.

"Lube," he says, "plenty of lube. That's really important."

I watch as he coats his fingertips with the glossy liquid.

"And we have to get you ready, first."

"Ready?"

"It helps if you're nice and relaxed. A good climax should do it."

My eyes light up. He isn't teasing me. He's going to let me come, right from the start. While I watch, heart racing, Charlie starts to touch me. After all this time, he knows perfectly well what turns me on. He rubs the ball of his thumb over my clit, and I groan. Then he begins to make those little circles, around and around, until my breathing starts to come more rapidly.

I watch him the whole time, feeling disbelief. Charlie never lets me come so quickly. But this is a stage that his manual has described. It's important for the woman to be ready. And ready to Charlie means this...

He spreads my pussy lips apart with both hands and then runs his thumbs over my clit. First one, then the other, until I am crying out. He starts soft and sweet at first, then begins to touch me more firmly, until I'm shaking the bed, my whole body trembling.

"Let yourself go," Charlie instructs, and I do, moaning aloud with the power of my climax, shuddering all over from the force of it. And immediately, Charlie gets that look in his eye. That Doctor of Love look. I'm ready—so he is ready. He moves closer to me, then starts to slide his hand into me, curving his fingers upward, as if trying to pull me up off the bed from within my body.

I shudder at the feeling, still reeling from my most recent climax.

"Is it there?" Charlie asks.

"What do you mean?"

"Is this the spot?"

I wasn't sure, which makes Charlie think he hasn't found the right location. "It should be just about two inches inside of you," he says, consulting his notes again. "And if I touch you right, you might feel as if you have to pee."

"That's doing it *right*?" I ask.

"The need will pass," he assures me. "If you can handle the feeling, work through it, I promise the urge will go away in a few seconds," and as he speaks, he seems to find what he is looking for. Or what I've been looking for. Because suddenly I feel something I've never felt before. It's crazy. I grip on to Charlie's wrist. "Right there," I say, whispering. "There."

"Here?" He continues to press, his fingers massaging the most perfect location. I can hardly believe the sensation. I've never felt anything like this before.

"You might bring your knees up to your chest," Charlie suggests, his fingers still curved, pulling up on me, pressing harder and harder. He moves his hand in the same rhythm as if he were fucking me, but his fingers are doing the work instead of his cock. I feel the pleasure, feel the wave of it build within me, and then suddenly I come. But this isn't just coming— not like I've climaxed in the past. This is like exploding, the pleasure ricocheting throughout my entire body.

"Oh, my god—" At first I think I've said it, but the words come from Charlie.

"Look at that!" he continues, and I realize his hand is covered with my liquid. "Did that feel as good as it looked?" he asks, bringing his body close to mine, so that I can feel his cock, hard against my thigh. The

Doctor of Love has clearly gotten aroused during his examination of me.

"Oh, yeah," I tell him, still finding speaking rather difficult.

"Did you know you could come like that?"

I shake my head.

"Just feel," he says, taking my own hands and putting them over my pussy. Letting me see how wet I've gotten, letting me trace my fingertips in my own ejaculate. I am shocked by the amount of fluid, and when I bring my hands back up to my face, I see traces of the milky liquid. Afterward, being as clinical an observer as he is, I ask him to get that mirror out again to show me my wet and dripping pussy lips.

But even a Doctor of Love has his limits. Charlie is on me next, fucking me fiercely, unable to stop himself. The whole time, he whispers to me how turned on I've made him. How my pleasure has fueled his own.

"I can't wait to try that again," he says. "But with my cock instead of my fingers."

It's fun dating someone who considers himself a Doctor of Love. Of course, I know the reality of what he is. But I'd never call him that to his face.

shopping and further study

Finding the right G-spot toy, book or video for adventure and further study takes both having an idea of what you might be looking for (or actually, looking to do), and finding a store that sells your item. It's important to determine your intentions in advance; know what you'd like your toy to do, and have a specific item in mind. The other half of the equation is finding a good place to shop, so be prepared to check out more than one store. Of course, you can do a lot of your shopping at one site, Amazon.com (and the prices are usually rockbottom), but that has its disadvantages too as you'll still have your items shipped from different stores within Amazon (different arrival times for your packages), and the quality will vary greatly from store to store. And don't expect these stores to have great return policies on broken items—it's a risk that can go either way.

If you're shopping in person, find a store that will be a comfortable place to shop. Almost all cities have a selection of adult toy, book, and video stores that are somewhat (or even very) sleazy and uncomfortable to visit, generally because they aren't clean or kept up in any visible way, and the customers and clerks don't seem to want to be seen there. These can be great places to find cheap G-spot toys, books and videos, though keep in mind that you'll likely see things in the store that'll totally turn you off or offend you—or will make you run from the store laughing. Often though, these stores are not so scary and you'll get what you want, pay the bored cashier (who's seen it all, by the way), and go home. Either way, it's highly recommended that before you buy anything online or in person, you and your lover make the trek to a store to see and handle the toys in person at least once so you both get a realistic idea of what you're buying (or not).

At women-oriented sex toy boutiques, you'll see a lot of other women and men shopping: people of every stripe and persuasion. Unfortunately these clean, well-lit places to shop for sex toys are found only in a few major cities, such as those noted in parentheses in the following list.

On websites, it's important to safeguard your privacy. Shop at reputable stores; if you're not sure about their reputation see if they have online forums where you can garner customer feedback, check to see if they have actual brick-and-mortar stores (a sign of stability), and Google their URL and name to see what you dig up. Check to see what their privacy policy is—if it's dodgy, shop elsewhere. See how they ship their products—is the process discreet and do the toys come in plain packages? And finally, see how their products are presented: if they have offensive or misspelled product descriptions or sell products that are unsafe, or if they just seem a bit off, then they'll likely treat their customers with the same disdain. Do they have annoying pop-up windows? Skip 'em. Shop with someone you like, and if they have an educational section or mission statement, even better.

Shopping Resources

Online and Mail Order

Babeland

Website, retail stores, and catalog of toys, books, videos, and safer-sex supplies. Women-owned and operated, but open to all orientations. Strict privacy policy. (For retail information, see the "Retail Stores" section below.)
800 658 9119
babeland.com

Blowfish

Mail-order catalog and website of toys, books, videos, DVDs, safer-sex supplies, S/M gear, comics, and magazines. They feature individual reviews of their products and a strict privacy policy.
P.O. Box 411290, San Francisco, CA 94141
800 325 2569
415 252 4340
blowfish.com

Coco de Mer

A sophisticated sex toy boutique founded by the daughter of Body Shop owner Anita Rod-

dick, their websites and stores in the UK and US feature smart selections and unique tools for enhancing fellatio. (For retail information, see "Retail Stores" below.)
020 7836 8882 (UK)
1 866 959 2626 (US)
coco-de-mer.com (UK)
cocodemerusa.com (US)

Condomania
Exhaustive site that sells virtually every condom under the sun, with fun facts, lots of condom information, and a helpful condom shopping guide.
1 800 9CONDOM
1 800 926 6366
condomania.com

Glyde Dams
Buy 'em here, by the dozen or in a party pack!
sheerglydedams.com

Good Vibrations
Good Vibrations has a staff who are committed to dispensing accurate sex information about the products they sell. Website and retail stores carry toys, books, and DVDs. (For retail

information, see the "Retail Stores" section below.)
934 Howard St., San Francisco, CA 94103
800 289 8423
415 974 8990
goodvibes.com

LoveHoney

This UK-based site is a one-stop shop for quality sex toys, books, and videos. They make their
own product videos, have an entertaining blog,
and are committed to green practices and environmentally conscious products.
100 Locksbrook Rd.
Bath, BA1 3EN
England
0800 915 6635
lovehoney.co.uk

Retail Stores

A Woman's Touch

Feminist sex store offering toys, books, and safer-sex supplies. Their website has great advice
columns.
600 Williamson St., Madison, WI 53703

608 250 1928
200 N. Jefferson St., Milwaukee, WI 53202
414 221 0400
888-621-8880
a-womans-touch.com

Babeland

Retail store, website, and catalog of high-quality, carefully selected toys, books, videos, and safer-sex supplies. Women-owned and operated, and open to all orientations. They have in-store educational workshops and a highly trained staff.

707 E. Pike St., Seattle, WA 98122
206 328 2914
94 Rivington St., New York, NY 10002
212 375 1701
43 Mercer St., New York, NY 10013
212 966 2120
462 Bergen St., Brooklyn, NY 11217
718 638 3820
(Mail order) 800 658 9119
babeland.com

Come Again Erotic Emporium

Woman-owned store with toys, books, and lingerie.

353 E. 53rd St., New York, NY 10022
212 308 9394

Eve's Garden

Woman-focused store with toys, books, and videos.
119 W. 57th St., 12th Floor, New York, NY 10019
800 848 3837
212 757 8651
evesgarden.com

Forbidden Fruit

Woman-owned and operated toy store/adult gift shop, and fetish boutique. A big supporter of the Austin S/M, fetish, safer-sex, and sex-positive communities.
108 E. North Loop Blvd., Austin, TX 78751
512-453-8090
www.forbiddenfruit.com

Good Vibrations

Staff is trained, and their Education department serves staff and customers and does outreach to health organizations. Website and retail stores carry toys, books, DVDs, safer-sex supplies.
603 Valencia St., San Francisco, CA 94110
415 522 5460

1620 Polk St., San Francisco, CA 94109
415 345 0400
899 Mission St., San Francisco, CA 94103
415 513 1635
2504 San Pablo Ave., Berkeley, CA 94702
510 841 8987
3219 Lakeshore Ave., Oakland, CA 94610
510 788 2389
308A Harvard St., Brookline, MA 02446
617 264 4400
(Mail Order) 800 289 8423
www.goodvibes.com
(See "Online and Mail Order" section for more mail order/Web info.)

Pleasure Chest

Retail store and website of novelties, toys, videos, and clothing.
7733 Santa Monica Blvd., West Hollywood, CA 90046
800 75 DILDO
323 650 1022
156 Seventh Ave. S., New York, NY 10014
212 242 2158
3436 N. Lincoln Ave., Chicago, IL 60657
773 525 7151
thepleasurechest.com

Canadian Resources

Come As You Are

No visit to Toronto is complete without visiting this community-oriented worker-owned co-op retail store, and they also have a mail-order catalog and website. They have toys, books, videos, safer-sex supplies, and educational resources, especially resources for the disabled. Products are hand-picked and individually reviewed. Stores offer educational workshops. *Nous offrons des services limites en francais.*

701 Queen St. W., Toronto, ON, M6J 1E6, Canada
(Toll-free) 888 504 7934
416 504 7934
comeasyouare.com

Good For Her

Woman-focused retail store carries toys, books, videos, and erotic art; hosts sex workshops, all geared toward female pleasure. In addition to regular hours, store has women and trans-only hours.

175 Harbord St., Toronto, ON, M5S 1H3, Canada
(Toll-free) 877 588 0900
416 588 0900
goodforher.com

Lovecraft

Retail stores and website offering toys, books, videos, and lingerie. Possibly the oldest women-owned sex shop in North America—open since 1972.

2200 Dundas St. E., Mississauga, ON, L4X 2V3, Canada

905 276 5772

(Toll-free) 877 923 7331

lovecraftsexshop.com

Womyn's Ware

Retail store, website, and catalog of toys, books, and fetish gear, education- and woman-focused. Store hosts sex seminars.

896 Commercial Dr., Vancouver, BC, V5L 3Y5, Canada

604 254 2543

(Toll-free) 888 996 9273

womynsware.com

European Resources

Le Boudoir

The Spanish woman's answer to a female-friendly, smart, and sexy online sex shopping experience—from Spain, they are a fabulous resource. Lovely; website is in Spanish.
leboudoir.net

LoveHoney

This UK-based site is a one-stop shop for quality sex toys, books, and videos. They make their own product videos, have an entertaining blog, and are committed to green practices and environmentally conscious products.
lovehoney.co.uk

Lust

A women-run, women-focused online sex boutique from Denmark, with a lovely site and fantastic selection. Site is in Danish.
lust.dk

Second Sexe

French website, erotic boutique, and resource for women positive, feminist-identified products and porn. Exquisite site, lots to choose from.

secondsexe.com

SH!

A women's sex shop that is all-inclusive and couples friendly, with two levels including handpicked toys, books, videos and lingerie. A well-educated staff, many after hours events and comfortable atmosphere.

57 Hoxton Square, London N1 6PB U.K.

Tel. 020 7613 5458

sh-womenstore.com

Tiberius

Austrian leather, latex and a variety of sexy tools.

A-1070 Wien, Lindengasse 2, Austria

Tel. 43 1 522 04 74

tiberius.at

leather@tiberius.at

Yoba

A gorgeous online women's sex toy boutique, with lingerie and their own beautiful sex magazine. I wish American sex toy boutiques looked and felt like this (site is in French).

yobaparis.com

Safer-Sex Resources

American Social Health Association
P.O. Box 13827, Research Triangle Park, NC 27709
919 361 8400
ashastd.org

Center for Disease Control National Prevention Information Network
P.O. Box 6003, Rockville, MD 20849
800 458 5231
cdcnpin.com

National AIDS Hotline
800 232 4636

National STI Resource Center Hotline
919 361 8488

Planned Parenthood
800 230 PLAN
plannedparenthood.org

Safer Sex Page
safersex.org

San Francisco Sex Information

Sex information and referral switchboard that provides free, nonjudgmental, anonymous, confidential, accurate information from a highly trained staff. Monday through Thursday 3:00 P.M. to 9:00 P.M.; Friday 3:00 P.M. to 6:00 P.M.; Sunday 2:00 P.M. to 5:00 P.M. PST. Ask any question about sex under the sun by emailing ask-us@sfsi.org.

415 989 SFSI

sfsi.org

Sex Education Classes and Workshops:

Organizations

(For stores near you that offer sex education workshops and classes, see the "Retail Stores" section.)

Body Electric

School of healing arts dedicated to exploring the healing potential of erotic energy, with a holistic, mindful, and spiritual approach (open to all spiritual orientations). Classes for men and for women, mixed classes, retreats, and more, in Seattle, Oakland, New York, and Los Angeles.

3771 Texas St., San Diego, CA 92104

510 653 1594
thebodyelectricschool.com

San Francisco Sex Information

Sex information and referral switchboard that
provides free, nonjudgmental, anonymous, accurate information. They offer a fifty-five-hour
training course in all aspects of human sexuality and monthly Continuing Education classes
open to the public on a variety of current topics;
for more information, see their website.
415 989 SFSI
sfsi.org

Society for Human Sexuality

Social and educational organization that offers
lectures and programs with the Center for Sex-
Positive Culture in Seattle. They have a huge online library of sex resources.
PMB 1276, 1122 E. Pike St., Seattle, WA 98122
sexuality.org

Sex-Related Websites

Cleis Press
Cleis has published groundbreaking, informative, and controversial books about sex and politics since 1980. The publisher of this book, they also have a great website showcasing their latest erotica, all their sex guidebooks, and Midnight Editions, their incredible consciousness-raising human rights books.
cleispress.com

G-Spot Center
gspotcenter.com

G-Spot Facts and Resources: Tiny Nibbles and Open Source Sex
Tiring of websites that are low on information and updated resources on the G-spot. I created this page on my website to serve as both a starting point and continuing education resource that includes podcasts, videos, erotica, articles on the G-spot, and more.
tinynibbles.com/gspot

G-Spot: Wikipedia
en.wikipedia.org/wiki/G-spot

GLBT National Hotline

The GLNH is an all-volunteer, nonprofit organization. They provide telephone info, email info, referrals, and peer counseling for the GLBT communities. They have over 18,000 listings for the entire US, including groups, organizations, business, bars, doctors, lawyers, therapists, etc. Monday through Friday 4:00 P.M. to midnight; Saturday noon to 5:00 P.M. EST.
888 THE GLNH, 888 843 4564
glbtnationalhelpcenter.org

Scarlet Letters

Webzine of articles, erotica, and more.
scarletletters.com

Scarleteen

Resource of sex information geared toward teen women, but with great sections for young men.
scarleteen.com

SIECUS (Sexuality Information and Education Council of the United States)

SIECUS is a national nonprofit organization that develops, collects, and disseminates information on sex, promotes sex education, and advocates individual choice.

90 John St., Ste. 402, New York, NY 10038
212 819 9770
1012 14th St., NW, Suite 107, Washington DC
20005
202 265 2405
siecus.org

Tiny Nibbles: Violet Blue's Open Source Sex

My own website for sex culture commentary, accurate sex information, updated resources for all things related to human sexuality, an awesome blog, and epicenter for current information on new sex books, sex videos, sex studies, sex in the news, my famous podcast, TV appearances, news on people doing cool things in the world of sex, and much, much more.
tinynibbles.com

The Sex Carnival

Run by a woman and staffed by several others, this multi-author sex blog is a resource bar none on sex toy reviews, sex news, sex classes, and most especially the world of kinky sex.
thesexcarnival.com

Highly Recommended Reading

The Clitoral Truth: The Secret World at Your Fingertips by Rebecca Chalker

Female Ejaculation and the G-Spot by Deborah Sundahl

The Good Vibrations Guide to the G-Spot by Cathy Winks

The G-Spot: And Other Discoveries About Human Sexuality by Alice Kahn Ladas, Beverly Whipple and John D. Perry

The Guide to Getting It On! by Paul Joannides

A Hand in the Bush: The Fine Art of Vaginal Fisting by Deborah Addington

The Survivor's Guide to Sex: How to Have an Empowered Sex Life After Childhood Sexual Abuse by Staci Haines

The Ultimate Guide to Anal Sex for Women by Tristan Taormino

The Ultimate Guide to Cunnilingus by Violet Blue

The Ultimate Guide to Orgasm for Women by Mikaya Heart

The Ultimate Guide to Sex and Disability by Miriam Kaufman, Cory Silverberg and Fran Odette

The Ultimate Guide to Sexual Fantasy by Violet Blue

The Ultimate Guide to Strap-On Sex by Karlyn Lotney

The Whole Lesbian Sex Book: A Passionate Guide for All of Us (2nd. Ed.) by Felice Newman

Recommended Viewing
(A caveat: it's difficult to find modern-looking videos on this topic.)

The Best of Vulva Massage, The New School of Erotic Touch

Unlocking the Secrets of G-Spot (DVD), Better Sex Video series, Sinclair Intimacy Institute

Female Ejaculation for Couples, Fatale Media

G Marks the Spot, Sexpositive Productions

How to Female Ejaculate: Find Your G-Spot, Fatale Media

Safe Sex Info
Before you put each other's naughty bits in your mouths or even think about rubbing your bodies together, it's a good idea to know where these bits have been. But since we don't all live in a perfect world—in fact, no one does—you'll want to use condoms, gloves, dental dams or finger cots when you have oral, vaginal and anal sex; when you use or share sex toys; and in some cases, when you give hand jobs. When someone pulls out a condom, dam, glove or 'cot, you know you're in good hands. Here are the items in your first line of defense against invading infections and viruses, in short order:

Condoms: Available in latex and polyurethane, in dozens of sizes, colors and flavors. Animal skin condoms do not prevent the spread of some viruses. A condom is a snug sheath that unrolls onto a penis or sex toy. Use condoms for fellatio, for vaginal and anal sex, for covering sex toys that are made of porous materials, or for when you want to share a sex toy. Change condoms for different sex partners and orifices—something used anally should be covered with a condom before being inserted orally or vaginally. Don't reuse your toy condoms. Do not use anything containing oils of any kind where latex condoms may come in contact; however, polyurethane condoms may be used with oils.

Dental Dams: Thin squares of latex or polyurethane used as barriers for cunnilingus and rimming. Lubricate the genitals, place the dam on top, keep a good hold on the dam and lick to your heart's content. Available in a few flavors and colors. In a jam you can use plastic wrap or a condom cut open and laid flat.

Gloves: Use latex or nonlatex gloves for hand jobs on any gender. They protect against germs from your hands going onto genitals, can protect your hands from picking up viruses or germs, and make hands a smooth surface free of jagged nails or scratchy calluses.

Finger Cots: Tiny condoms made of latex that unroll over a finger to create a sterile surface. Great for on-the-go escapades.

If you choose to go at it uncovered, here is what you are at risk for. Make an informed decision!

Sharing Sex Toys

HIGH RISK	MODERATE RISK	NO RISK	N/A
Chlamydia	Bacterial vaginosis	None	None
Gonorrhea	Hepatitis A		
Hepatitis B	Hepatitis C		
HIV	Herpes		
Syphilis	HPV		
	Lice/scabies		
	Vaginitis		

Anal to Oral Contact (Penis or Sex Toy)

HIGH RISK	MODERATE RISK	NO RISK	N/A
Gonorrhea	HIV	Lice/scabies	Bacterial vaginosis
Hepatitis A	Chlamydia		Vaginitis
Hepatitis B	Hepatitis C		
Herpes			
HPV			
Syphilis			

Unprotected Anal to Vaginal Contact

HIGH RISK	MODERATE RISK	NO RISK	N/A
Bacterial vaginosis	Hepatitis C		Lice/scabies
Chlamydia			
Gonorrhea			
Hepatitis A			
Hepatitis B			
Herpes			
HIV			
HPV			
Syphilis			

about the author

VIOLET BLUE (tinynibbles.com, @violetblue) is a CBSi/ZDNet columnist, a *Forbes* "Web Celeb" and one of *Wired*'s "Faces of Innovation"—in addition to being a blogger, high-profile tech personality and podcaster. Violet has nearly forty award-winning, best-selling books; an excerpt from her *Smart Girl's Guide to Porn* is featured on Oprah Winfrey's website. She is regarded as the foremost expert in the field of sex and technology, a sex-positive pundit in mainstream media (CNN, "The Oprah Winfrey Show," "The Tyra Banks Show") and is regularly interviewed, quoted and featured prominently by major media outlets. Blue also writes for media outlets such as *MacLife, O: The Oprah Magazine* and the UN-sponsored international health organization RH Reality Check. She headlines at conferences ranging from ETech, LeWeb and SXSW: Interactive, to Google Tech Talks at Google, Inc. The *London Times* named Blue "one of the 40 bloggers who really count."

"Ultimate" Sex Guides

The Ultimate Guide to Fellatio
How to Go Down on a Man and Give
Him Mind-Blowing Pleasure
Violet Blue

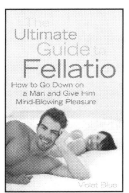

From talking to your partner about fellatio to male pleasure spots and sexual response, Violet Blue covers rimming, shaving, positions, oral sex games for couples, flavored lubricants, sex toys, and a plethora of oral techniques.
ISBN 978-1-57344-398-2 $16.95

The Ultimate Guide to Anal Sex for Men
Bill Brent

The complete guide for all men—heterosexual, gay, and bisexual—who want to experience the pleasure of anal sex.
ISBN 978-1-57344-121-6 $16.95

The Ultimate Guide to Adult Videos
How to Watch Adult Videos and Make Your Sex Life Sizzle
Violet Blue

The most complete resource for enjoying adult videos and DVDs. Packed with games, advice for couples and first-time viewers, and over 300 reviews of adult films. "Worth reading, worth buying, worth keeping."—Mike Ostrowski, *Playboy*
ISBN 978-1-57344-172-8 $16.95

The Ultimate Guide to Sexual Fantasy
How to Turn Your Fantasies into Reality
Violet Blue

Turn your favorite sexual fantasies into reality, safely and successfully... The complete guide for everyone—women and men, singles and couples!
ISBN 978-1-57344-190-2 $15.95

The Ultimate Guide to Anal Sex for Women
Tristan Taormino
Expanded and Updated Second Edition

Recommended by the *Playboy* Advisor and *Loveline*—the only self-help book on anal sex for women. "A book that's long overdue!...informative, sexy, and inspirational."—Betty Dodson
ISBN 978-1-57344-221-3 $16.95

Ordering is easy! Call us toll free or fax us to place your MC/VISA order.
You can also mail the order form below with payment to:
Cleis Press, 2246 Sixth St., Berkeley, CA 94710.

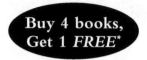

ORDER FORM

QTY	TITLE	PRICE

	SUBTOTAL	
	SHIPPING	
	SALES TAX	
	TOTAL	

Add $3.95 postage/handling for the first book ordered and $1.00 for each additional book. Outside North America, please contact us for shipping rates. California residents add 8.75% sales tax. Payment in U.S. dollars only.

* Free book of equal or lesser value. Shipping and applicable sales tax extra.

**Cleis Press • Phone: (800) 780-2279 • Fax: (510) 845-8001
orders@cleispress.com • www.cleispress.com
You'll find more great books on our website**

Follow us on Twitter @cleispress • Friend/fan us on Facebook

Printed in the United States
By Bookmasters